Jan 2021

J0695776

Copyright © 2015 by Pete Huttlinger
and Erin Morris Huttlinger

All rights reserved. In accordance with
the U.S. Copyright Act of 1976.

The scanning, uploading, and electronic sharing of any part of this
book without the permission of the publisher constitue unlawful
piracy and theft of the author's intellectual property.
If you would like to use material from the book (other than for review purposes), prior written permission must be obtained by con-
tacting the publisher at instar@petehuttlinger.com

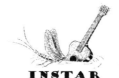

Instar Publishing
P.O. Box 58283
Nashville, TN 37205
www.petehuttlinger.com

First edition: July 2015
ISBN 978-0-692-43626-4

Book design and cover by Antsy McClain
Back cover photo courtesy of Lance Atchison
Benefit photos courtesy of Dan Harr

JOINED

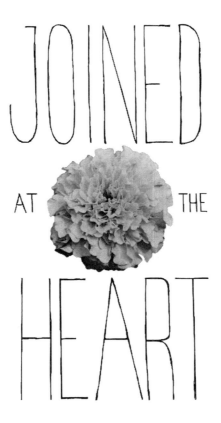

AT THE

HEART

A story of love, guitars,
resilience and marigolds

Pete Huttlinger &
Erin Morris Huttlinger

Foreword by John Oates

Dedication

This book is dedicated to the strongest children in the world, Sean and James; to our families who are precious and indispensable; to our friends all over the world whose love permeates our lives every day; and to Dr. Frank Fish who is literally a life saver many times over, and the best friend a heart patient could ever have.

Acknowledgements

It isn't that our memories are short or our gratitude less than profound when we declare that there are simply too many doctors, nurses, researchers and social workers involved in saving Pete's life and my happiness to thank here. There were dozens of them, and if we reproduced the entire personnel directories of Vanderbilt University Medical Center, Texas Heart Institute and Stanford University Hospital, there would still be some vital people we unforgivably left out. So rather than endlessly listing, we propose this instead: If you were among this legion of ministering angels, every time you see Pete play or hear his records or watch his videos, say to yourself and to anyone around you, 'I made that happen."

It's true, you know, and we'll swear to it.

Contents

Foreword

Around 2006 I was preparing to record my second solo album. It was the first time I would be recording in Nashville. My guide to the studios was the legendary engineer Bil Vorndick. He was well established in town and seemed to know everyone. At some point during the recording, he suggested I meet a gal named Erin Morris, a publicist and "in the know" person, to help get the word out on my first Nashville project.

Erin and I began to work together, and her network reached deep into the music community. In the course of getting to know each other, I found out that she was married to a very remarkable guitarist named Pete Huttlinger. Pete was world famous for his finger picking prowess and his work with John Denver, among others. I had a connection to John Denver, having seen him play in 1968 at a small bar in Snowmass Colorado. Besides that, we both lived in Aspen and had been label mates on RCA Records in the 1970s.

Pete and Erin had many ties in Colorado, where I was living at the time. On one of their trips west, we met for lunch near my house at a local watering hole called the Woody Creek Tavern. Pete was booked to play that evening at Steve's Guitars, a very cool living room style venue in a Victorian house in the small town of Carbondale. He asked me if I wanted to come and perhaps sit in. I recall us hanging out before the show in the little up-stairs office that served as a dressing room. We messed around with a few Doc Watson tunes, and my first impression was that while I was attending fingerpicking class 101, Pete was more on the Ph. D. I have always loved playing with great players, and we hit it off that night which led to us traveling around the country playing and recording together in the following years.

When I first heard the news about his stroke, needless to say I was shocked and saddened to think of the very real possibility that such an immense talent might be silenced so suddenly and completely. From afar, I tried to keep up with his recovery, which culminated in the day he returned to the hospital that treated him to astound the doctors by playing for them in record time. The trials and almost overwhelming medical and personal challenges that lay ahead will be better described in the pages to follow.

This is a story of overcoming seemingly impossible odds, passion, friendship, guts and the ultimate affirmation of the human spirit. I am proud to know Erin and Pete and bear witness to their strength and success.

– John Oates

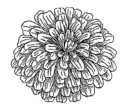

*S*oul mates, being a team, sweethearts, lovers... there are so many phrases used to describe the perfect combination of two people who are in love. I've tried to think of something uniquely our own to put into words what I think is the most amazing, loving relationship I could have. I can't come up with a phrase, but I can come up with a visual. Picture two objects. They are different shades of the same color. They are similar, but not exactly the same shape. The objects are bright and move quickly and steadily. They are always within reach of each other and move amazingly synchronized through the air. They come together and they move apart, but they always are within range of each other. They compensate exactly within perfect ratio of what one needs and the other has to offer. One never gets larger than or overshadows the other. They never harm each other.

They share a heartbeat.

Chapter One

The Point

B oth as a team and as a married couple, we have always worked with specific "destinations" in mind. Where are we going professionally and personally, we ask ourselves, and what are the best routes for getting there? We're workaholics because we love our jobs—Pete as a world-class guitarist and Erin as a publicist for such world-renowned musicians as Vince Gill, Waylon Jennings, Martina McBride, Alabama, and many others. And we're family-holics, too, because our families are genuinely fascinating people (in so many strange and wonderful ways).

Because we are destination-oriented, that's how we've approached writing this book. What point do we want to make, and what life-stories do we need to tell to make it? Well, our point is simply to encourage people who are facing adversity to summon up the love, energy and stamina it takes not just to live but to live well.

As a couple that's lived on the edge of death and despair—not once but often—and survived to celebrate life, we urge you to embrace life as long as even a flicker remains and to help others do the same. We encourage you to pull yourself from the depths of whatever your personal trauma is and realize that it can be the beginning of a joyful life. In our case, our depths were health related. But we've discovered that love and determination eases calamity in all its forms.

As we were going through our tough times (which by no means have ended), people often told us that they were inspired by our love and persistence. In all honesty, we didn't see ourselves that way. Quite frankly, we were a little embarrassed to get so much credit for what we felt was just natural, honest behavior. We're still not sure that our conduct was anything more than that, but enough people have encouraged us to tell our story that we thought we should perk up our ears and listen to them.

If your family says you have a story to tell, you take it with a grain of salt. If family and friends both say it, it's motivating but still not altogether persuasive. But if your family, friends and wonderful fans from around the world all insist that your story is inspiring, then there must be something to it.
So here is our story.

Pete Huttlinger   *Erin Morris Huttlinger*

Chapter Two

The Connection

Erin

Many years ago when we started working together Pete informed me, his then very confused manager, "I have a bad heart and one day it will just wear out." That phrase has rung in my ears for many years.

Pete and I met in 1998 at a John Denver tribute show in Aspen, Colorado. Pete toured as part of John's phenomenal band for many years. And beginning in 1998, one year after John's

3

tragic death in a plane crash, a number of his band mates, family, friends and fans from around the world, gathered in Aspen to mourn his death and celebrate his life. It was at the very first one of these gatherings that Pete and I crossed paths. I had been invited to handle the public relations for the concert and Pete was there as a performer. I watched him work in rehearsals and perform for two nights. He was a serious musician, a perfectionist and a leader. Sometimes he seemed too rough in his direction of the rest of the band, or at least that is what I thought. I was not accustomed to the back and forth between band members during rehearsals. We laugh about it now, how my first impression of him couldn't have been more wrong.

I have lived and worked in Nashville since 1981. I started at Billboard magazine (the industry's leading trade publication) and was recruited by RCA Records for their public relations department in 1984. I was still a senior in college. During my RCA tenure I was fortunate to have worked with some of the greatest performers of all time. From Waylon Jennings to Dolly Parton, Vince Gill, Kenny Rogers, Alabama, The Judds, Roy Rogers, Bill Medley, Clint Black, Restless Heart, Martina McBride – an endless list of country music royalty. After 11 years with RCA in positions that ranged from Product Manager to head of Public Relations for the Nashville division, I was pregnant with my second child and decided it was time to leave. The travel was demanding and with a 2-year-old and another on the way, I needed to be home a little bit more. So I left the security of the corporate world and joined my now ex-husband at our own PR agency. I have worked for myself ever since.

Following that weekend, Pete and I began working together — a team in the most perfect sense of the word — initially as his publicist, eventually as his manager, and ultimately as his wife.

Since 1998 I have been aware of his congenital defect. And even during the years when there were no really obvious effects, I was always watching him--worrying about him. Keeping my eyes peeled for anything that wasn't right. I am certain that there were times when this was annoying to him, but he never said so. I believe that he always appreciated the fact that I truly cared for him whether it was as his manager or as his wife.

His deterioration over the last twelve years was incredibly gradual. During this time we have toured extensively, hiked, fly-fished and have flown in and out of cities in nearly every state in the nation and around the world. He is a high energy guy that likes to work hard, work fast, accomplish a lot and play his guitar for hours every day. There would be no clue to an outsider that there was ever anything wrong with him. And as his manager I tried to make sure that nobody that we worked with ever knew what was going on, partly because they would treat him differently and partly because they might not want to book him as a performer. As time went on I brought some of the people we worked with on a regular basis in on what his condition was. Eventually I had to let everyone know. The main side effect of his condition was that he would tire, and when he did he had to rest. Not an option. It also affected his ability to lift and carry his equipment, suitcases and guitars. So slowly but surely, the environment we worked in became aware of his somewhat fragile situation. And every single friend, promoter, peer and fan have been sincerely supportive. I think this is a testament to the mission that Pete and I have had since we first began working together. We agreed to work under the theory that we wanted to leave a good taste in everyone's mouth. Whether it is the usher in the theater, the cab driver, the promoter, the journalist, the fan in the front row or the fan in the back row, they will be treated with respect and appreciation and made to feel like they are part of our team. That mission served us well, but we had no idea just how well it would serve us.

Pete

I was born at 8:31 AM on June 22nd at Columbia Women's Hospital in Washington D.C. My father, Joseph B. Huttlinger Sr. phoned our home and word quickly spread to my sister, Theresa (T), who was 13 and my brothers Mike 11, Joe Jr. 7, Carl 5 and Frank 2 that I might not be coming home from the hospital. They got word that the new baby was sick. There was something wrong with his heart and he might not be strong enough to come home… ever.

I like to think that there was a sadness that came over the room at home that day. But in reality there were five children at home and they had other things to worry about:

Who took my candy bar? I want to know and I want to know now.

Where's my toy jet?

Does this dress look pretty?

Can I have some milk?

Hey, look! I pooped in the toilet.

WHERE'S MY CANDY BAR?

They were no more thinking about me than I was about them. I was just lying lazily in the hospital. Sleeping, crying, feeding and trying desperately to breathe. But even in my desperation for a breath of air, I'm certain I was as relaxed as I could be. I don't ever want to put out anyone else for my own comfort. It's just not my style. I'm never as comfortable when someone does something for me, as I am when I am able to do something for them. I think we are born with that trait or not. I was one of the lucky ones to be born with it.

I was a blue baby. Kind of a funny term for a guy who is anything but blue. Even in the worst of times I find myself cracking a joke to make those around me feel at ease. But blue I was when I came out of the womb and the doctor knew immediately he had a problem on his hands.

My mom had had several miscarriages and lost two children (both sons) as infants before I was born. T would have been the eldest child and only girl in a family with eight kids, had my brothers who had been born earlier survived. At one point when mom went off to the hospital and the phone call came at the house from Dad that it was another boy, T was rumored to have said, "Oh, dad! Couldn't we have a turtle instead?"

I suppose a turtle would have been okay for a while but like all pets she would eventually outgrow it and it would lose its charm for her and hers would be lost for the turtle as well.

I was born with a fairly rare congenital heart defect. The actual condition is called:

Complex congenital heart disease with atrial-visceral situs inversus, atrioventricular and ventriculoarterial discordance, resulting in "mirror image" congenitally-corrected transposition. I was also born with an ASD (Atrial Septal Defect) and a VSD (Ventricular Septal Defect) and a pulmonary stenosis.

All those words combined mean that I was in terrible condition when it came to my heart's ability to pump blood throughout my body. Like Gilligan and the rest of the castaways' journey after their boat crashed on the rocks, my life would be an uphill climb.

Situs-Inversus with dextrocardia means that my organs are all reversed. So my heart is on the right side of my chest. My liver and gall bladder are on the left side of my abdomen and my stomach and spleen are on the right. My lungs are also reversed. The left side is my trilobed one and the right sided one is bilobed.

The ASD (Atrial Septal Defect) and VSD (Ventricular Septal Defect) refer to two specific defects in the heart. One in the atria and the other in the ventricles. These defects, or holes between the chambers, allow blood to flow where it shouldn't between the atria and the ventricles instead of to and from them. Normally, the right and left atria are separated by a septum called the interatrial septum. If this septum is defective, then oxygen-rich blood can flow directly from the left side of the heart to mix with the oxygen-poor blood in the right side of the heart, or vice versa. The result is called ASD.

A VSD refers to the ventricular septum, the wall dividing the right and left ventricles of the heart. Some of the blood from the left ventricle leaks into the right ventricle passes through the lungs and re-enters the left ventricle through the pulmonary veins and left atrium. The result of this is two-fold: volume overload on the left ventricle and pulmonary hypertension. None of this is good.

Obstruction of flow of blood from the right ventricle to the pulmonary artery results in what is called pulmonary stenosis.

Well, as luck would have it, they took me home from the hospital and though "thrive" might not be the right word, I got along okay. Trips to the doctor's office were regular. Shots were given to me every Thursday up until the age of five. Once, I remember hiding under a bed in our home to avoid getting a shot. T found me and told me matter-of-factly that I was going to have to get the shot either way. If not that day then it would be the next. She reminded me that I'd get a lollipop from the doctor. So always a sucker for logic, I crawled out from under the bed and we went to the doctor's office only to find out that it was the wrong day. Hallelujah!

My dad died when I was three years old and two years later we moved to California so mom could be near her family -- her support system. Her brothers and sisters and what seemed like truckloads of their kids all lived out there.

When I was twelve years old I entered junior high school. It's the first year the boys have to "dress down." You are required to get a jock strap and put it on in the gym. So I showed up with mine, put it on and my gym shorts over it. The coach then told us to go out, run a lap and meet him back at the trailer for instructions on whatever game we were to play. I was very concerned. I had not told anyone at school of my heart condition. Very few of my friends knew of it and the coach definitely did not know.

So off we went jogging around the quarter mile track. I made it exactly half way. My head got dizzy. My knees buckled and I hit the dirt. The other kids kept on running and I felt like a loser but I knew there was nothing I could do to change the situation. So after I caught my breath, I walked the other half of the track and went to the coach and told him that I had a bad heart. He told me to sit out the rest of the activities for that day and I was more than happy to do just that.

That night when I got home my mom asked how things went at school. I never wanted to alarm her but I knew that the school hadn't called her and that I should tell her. So reluctantly I said,

"Well mom... you remember that issue with my heart?"

"Yes, dear, I do."

"Well, I had a little teeny weeny incident today at school."

"Oh, tell me what happened."

She never, ever became alarmed when she was receiving bad news. She would take it in and then calmly respond. This time was no exception. She thanked me for telling her, handed me a note she'd written for me to give to the coach the next day and that was that.

The next thing I knew I was being hauled off to a hospital in San Francisco to have some tests done. They did a cardiac test with a catheter to my heart. Then I was sent to Stanford University Medical Center where we met Dr. Norman E. Shumway. He was a very famous doctor in the heart transplant world. He was not considering me for a transplant but for a surgical procedure to repair the ASD, VSD and stenosis. He suggested June. I said I thought that February would be better. He said he didn't want me to miss any school. I told him that would not be a problem. I was a normal twelve year old and I really didn't want to have to go to school. He won.

Six months later I was in the hospital in Palo Alto, California at Stanford getting prepped for surgery. In those days they shaved you from your neck down to your toes leaving only the hair on top of your head on your body. I was two weeks away from turning thirteen and had a full crop of pubic hair growing in nicely. They shaved it all off. I lay in bed, looked under the sheets and cried. It took me thirteen years to grow that. Would it take another thirteen to grow back? Can't we just forget about the surgery and let me and my baldness go home. I was mortified.

The next morning I was awakened by a nurse who told me that she was waking me up in order to give me a shot to put me to sleep. As a fan of comedy shows I immediately saw the humor in this Three Stooges type of situation, the one where the three of them are sleeping in bed. One of them snores too loudly. Another one wakes him and tells him, "Hey, wake up and go back to sleep."

I told the nurse that I was doing just fine sleeping before they woke me. She didn't laugh.

She also told me that my mom had phoned in to say that she slept through her alarm and that she wouldn't be able to make it before my surgery. I knew how tired she was. We lived over an hour away from the hospital and she'd been driving to and from it for the past three days. Plus there were others at home who needed her. I was a little sad but I also felt a great compassion for her even in that moment.

Now, as an adult, I could not imagine the guilt I would feel if I had to phone in my love for my child who was about to undergo heart surgery. She must have been devastated at the thought of her youngest having open heart surgery and she wasn't there to see him off. Not there to tell him she loved him.

But she was there when I came out of surgery. I remember when they woke me up. I couldn't speak because of the tube down my throat. So mom said, "Hi honey. I'm here. Wiggle your toes if you love mom." I wiggled them and went back to sleep. Mom was there and all was going to be well.

The next couple of weeks post-surgery went well and when I was released I asked Dr. Shumway a question. "Can I run?" I wanted to be able to run so badly and I never could. He looked down at me and said simply, "Listen to your body. It will tell you what you can do."

For the next 25 years I took Dr. Shumway's advice, listened to my body, and I lived a relatively healthy life. No hospital stays, no regular doctors' visits, very few checkups even. I hiked, swam, kayaked, biked, and even ran like a normal, healthy person.

Erin

It's important at this point in our story to explain what type of guitarist and performer Pete is in order to grasp what he lost and is working to regain.

Pete has played guitar since he was 14. Inspired by so many people in his life, he decided to go to Berklee College of Music in Boston in 1981. In 1984 he moved to Nashville and has made his living as a musician and performer ever since -- initially as a side-man for various Nashville-based shows and bands, and eventually as a touring member of John Denver's band. John was well known for surrounding himself with some of the most talented musicians in the business. Before John died in 1997, Pete was composing and recording his own music and had already released his first album. After John's death Pete evolved into a solo entertainer and less of a side-man although he has continued to work with such artists as LeAnn Rimes, John Oates (of Hall & Oates) and many others.

As a solo artist Pete has accomplished great things. In 2000 he was named National Fingerpick Champion and his solo career took off. He has become world renowned for his unique style of composing and performing acoustic fingerstyle guitar. He is known for his precision and speed and musicality. He is a player that a lot of other players admire and due to that type of notoriety he was signed as the first artist to Steve Vai's label, Favored

Nations Acoustic. Steve himself is a world renowned electric player and famous for being part of Frank Zappa's "Mothers Of Invention" and the metal band Whitesnake. As Steve once told me, "Pete is a world-class player. He does things on guitar that nobody else can do."

Pete was invited to perform at several of Eric Clapton's Crossroads Festivals and has performed at Carnegie Hall three times. He's been written about extensively and his work is critically acclaimed. To date he has nearly 10 albums along with numerous instructional DVDs and books.

Pete's fan base is world-wide and they are devoted.

Pete

Our life together was pretty swell before I got sick. We would travel a lot for my gigs. We went to Italy three or four times, Switzerland, France, England. We toured all over the US. We made a lot of great friends in almost every city we went to. We learned to cook, went to art museums and studied Italian. I went fly fishing in Switzerland, skied in the Italian Alps, hiked and fly fished in England. We spent a week in Alaska fishing and playing music. I teach at a lot of guitar camps. From Alaska to California to Ohio and points in between and beyond, I would show up with guitar in hand and a joke at the ready. I was very active to say the least.

At home we were just as busy. Spending time with Erin's kids, Sean and James, doing yard work, taking long walks in the neighborhood, hiking, canoeing all while keeping business rolling. Writing new music, publishing guitar instructional DVDs and books of my transcriptions from my CDs and finally recording new CDs.

Erin and I have always loved what we do for a living and having someone to share that love with who understands the passion and the drive that it takes to be really good at something is special.

Chapter Three

Copper Mountain

Erin

Our trip in August of 2010 to perform at a festival in Copper Mountain, CO was the first really traumatizing event where I could see the beginning of the end. Where I knew that we weren't getting off lightly anymore. It was my first time having to think clearly and quickly as to what to do in an emergency. Laughable now....it was just a warm up.

We were headed to Colorado. One of our favorite spots. We always look forward to flying into Denver then driving into the mountains. Every year we would make three or four trips out there to do shows. This particular trip was taking us to Copper

Mountain for a big guitar festival—Guitar Town, which was promoted by our good friend Bob Burwell, who is also manager for music legend Kenny Rogers and rock guitar god Steve Vai. The festival was at the base of the mountain.

Pete, only a few weeks prior, had had a pacemaker/defibrillator implanted. As with everything else involving Pete's anatomy, it was no piece of cake. Often an outpatient type of surgery, Pete's took over five hours as the doctors weaved wires (leads) around his reversed anatomy. Frankly, anyone could use additional oxygen at that elevation but Pete in particular needed it.

Pete

The first time I went to Copper Mountain to perform and teach at Bob's festival I was awe struck by the sheer size of the mountain. We pulled up shortly after sundown but the mountain was still visible. I remember standing outside the car and taking in a deep breath and staring at the mountain. What a beautiful place, I thought to myself. I couldn't wait to wake up the next morning to check it all out. I wanted to hike and see all the sights, maybe rent a bike and take to the trails.

I absolutely love being in the mountains. Whether they are in California or Tennessee, North Carolina, Virginia or Colorado I really don't care. I just love being outside and walking with a piece of straw hanging out of my mouth and soaking in the beauty around me.

I was born in Washington D.C and moved to California when I was five years old. In D.C. we would go to the beach to a place called Plumb Point on the Chesapeake Bay. But in California we would go to the mountains and I loved the mountains so much more. I can remember being very young and trying to keep up with my brothers in the Sierra's. I never minded not being able to keep up because I would stop and throw rocks or just smell the pines or stare at a creek for half an hour.

2010 was my second trip out to perform and teach at Guitar Town. Bob and I walked in and he carried my bags up the single flight of stairs. It didn't seem like much to me but almost as soon as we got to the top of the stairs Bob looked at me and said simply but matter-of-factly, "Sit down, right now." I looked at him and laughed and said, "What?" He said it again, "Sit down right now. I don't want you going down on me and you are about to go down." I wasn't sure what he was talking about but I sat down. He handed me a bottle of water and a granola bar and told me to eat and drink.

Copper Mountain, Colorado sits at approx. 9,712 feet. It's fair to say 10,000 feet because like my friend Jim Wood says "If something costs me $9.95 it's eaten up the best part of ten dollars, so I just say it cost me ten dollars." What's a few hundred feet when you are talking about nine thousand and seven hundred feet? So I just say ten thousand feet.

The oxygen level in the air at that altitude is quite low compared to the 400 - 1,000 feet around my home in Nashville, Tennessee. Combine that lower oxygen level with a congenital heart defect which has your health steadily declining for the past few years and you've got Bob Burwell telling you to "Sit down, right now!" because you are pale and breathing hard and you don't even notice because it's been coming on so slowly.

So there I sat while Bob (no youngster himself) checked us both in and immediately ordered an oxygen tank for me. It turned out that they had had some big event going on the weekend before and hadn't replenished all of their oxygen yet so they took one out of Duane Eddy's room (Yes, that Duane Eddy. Rock guitar legend and Hall Of Famer) and brought it to me. Duane hadn't arrived yet and I needed some oxygen so… This has been a running joke with me and Bob ever since. "Hey Pete," he says, "You took Duane Eddy's oxygen. Duane Eddy's! How does that make you feel?" "Well Bob, at the time… pretty darned good!" I guess survival of the fittest sometimes means survival of the first to arrive.

From the minute I arrived I was not feeling good. I slept with the oxygen on and I tossed and turned all night —woke up in the morning, took it off and got in the shower only to find myself breathless as soon as I stepped out. So the oxygen was back on for most of the remainder of the day except for when I would leave my room to get something to eat.

I didn't feel like eating anything but I knew I needed to. So I went to a local market, bought some Ramen noodles (Whoopee!) and I tried to eat them but they sucked. They seemed so simple and I used to love them 25 years earlier when I was in college. But when you're not feeling good and you can't breathe, Ramen noodles suck! Everything was horrible. I drank lots and lots of water because when you are at high altitude and it's so doggone dry, you need water. So I continued to drink and drink… and that was actually a big part of my next problem. When you have congestive heart failure and your heart is enlarged, water and salt are your number one and number two enemies. Ramen noodles are loaded with salt and I was drinking too much water.

I stayed in my room most of the day and all night, just trying to feel good but I was fading fast in spite of having the oxygen turned way up. My ever-expanding heart was growing larger by the minute it seemed.

The next day was the first day I had to work. I was teaching a class of guitar students, many of them had returned from the previous year, and I was excited to get started. When I got to the room where I was to teach I was completely out of breath. I had walked maybe 200 yards carrying my guitar and I was elated to see that Bob had had oxygen delivered to my teaching room. I sucked down on that mask rather quickly then began teaching. As the class went on I would occasionally grab the mask and I remember one lady in the class commenting that the altitude was a little tough but that I shouldn't be in need of so much oxygen. There was a little sound in her voice that sounded like she was implying that I was just being a wimp. I told that I had a heart condition and that I was indeed having a hard time breathing at this altitude.

Erin

Pete mentioned to me, more than once, that he didn't think the oxygen was helping him. It was obvious that he moved very slowly and seemed like a clock winding down. On Friday, the day before his concert, he released his students for their lunch break. As we walked to a local restaurant Pete kept slowing down. He told me, Sean my daughter who was also there to perform at the festival, and a couple of students, to go ahead to the restaurant and to not walk with him. He would catch up to us. I wasn't comfortable with that but I didn't want him to feel embarrassed that he was moving at a snail's pace.

There were five of us who sat down at a wonderful outside café facing the Copper Mountain ski run. It was a beautiful day. Pete was very quiet. Certainly not his energetic and talkative self. I felt anxious and worried. Our food came and as soon as Pete took his first bite, he began sobbing. Huge sobs. "I can't breathe," he said more than once. I thought to myself, "That's it. He's got to get off this mountain or he's going to die." Sean looked shocked as did the others at our table. They didn't know what to do or how to help. I told him to sit tight. Fortunately, Bob was within sight. I ran to him and told him what was going on. He knew Pete well enough to know that he wouldn't want to cancel an appearance. So he walked up to him and said, "Dude, you're outta here. I'm firing you." Bob threw me his car keys and said "Get him into Denver."

Pete sat while Sean and I rushed up to the room to grab his guitar and his bags. Joe Robinson, an amazing young guitarist, was assigned to finish teaching Pete's classes. We got him loaded into the car and I high-tailed it off that mountain as fast as I could. The pressure on Pete's lungs improved significantly every few hundred feet we came down. We called ahead to our friends Wes and Penny Weaver who lived on the close side of Denver. They were ready and waiting when we arrived. Pete was breathing significantly easier now so disaster seemed to be averted.

I was sad to leave him but knew he was in good hands. I had to return to Copper to be with Sean who did have to perform both that night and the next day. She was 18 and needed her "momager" with her for such a large event.

The drive back up to Copper was almost relaxing. I truly felt that Pete was now fine and would be fine until I could get back there on Sunday. I remember stopping at a Starbucks, getting an ice cold drink and just driving in silence and peace back up the mountain. I don't think I was actually relaxed, but it was such a distinctly different feeling than the previous two hours that it felt wonderful. The adrenaline was subsiding and it was so beautiful driving in the mountains.

After I returned and updated all of our friends and answered the fans' questions, I could relax and watch my daughter perform. Pete had checked in to wish her luck and said that he was resting and going to watch a movie with Wes and Penny. Sean's performance was wonderful and people were so kind to tell me how much they enjoyed the show. Fans for the next day's shows were arriving and I spent a lot of time explaining that Pete wasn't doing well and that I'd had to take him back into Denver. All of his fans— our friends really—were so understanding and concerned.

Pete

Wes, Penny and I were sitting down stairs at their home and were preparing to watch a movie. I was having a hard time catching my breath again. As the movie started I realized that I was in trouble again and I said, "Wes, how far is the hospital from your house?" "You need to go?" he asked. I told him I did and eleven minutes later we had completed a sixteen minute drive and I was in the emergency room. Wes said that he was certain that I was dehydrated and that they were going to get some fluids in me and I'd be good as gold.

As it turned out Wes' problem solving could not have been farther off the mark. After a quick evaluation, they inserted an IV in my arm and loaded me up with a drug called Lasix. It makes you urinate a lot and it works fast. It causes your body to rid itself of fluid built up in the lungs and around your heart. I'd had it one time before in Nashville and it's amazing how good you feel when you get rid of all that fluid that's built up. I think I filled two big jugs that they make you pee in before they sent me to a room.

I had the usual doctor's reaction to my condition when they

don't know me or are not already aware of my rare defect. Their eyebrows raise, they scratch their chins, tilt their heads and ask a bunch of questions — and then tell me that they'll be back. Eventually, they return and say they are going to admit me for further tests. This is the tell-tale sign that they don't yet have a clue what they are dealing with. These are the reactions I've gotten my whole life from doctors who are not involved with me personally.

Erin

Following the show Sean and I were having dinner with a couple of journalists that were covering the event when my phone rang. It was Pete. He said, "Don't worry but I'm on my way to the hospital." I felt sick. He told me he'd been struggling to breathe and Wes and Penny were rushing him to the hospital.

All through the night I was on the phone with his doctors at Swedish Hospital in Denver and Pete's cardiologist Dr. Frank Fish's team at Vanderbilt University Medical Center in Nashville. I was trying to make sure that everyone was talking to everyone and more importantly that they were listening to each other. They were. I tried to stay calm as did Sean. We watched television and tried to laugh. Pete was in good hands and there was nothing I could do. It wasn't a life or death situation as best I could tell, so I stayed with Sean through the next evening so she could perform.

Pete

The next day in my hospital room, I discovered the best food at any hospital in the world. I had grilled salmon with a honey glaze, fresh green beans and really tasty rice. They proved to me that it is possible to cook low-salt food and have it taste great! Unlike every other hospital I've been in throughout my life. They always serve things that look a lot like foods that one would normally eat at home. Chicken. Beef. Soups. Rice. Beans. Even desserts. Every hospital makes them and all but one ruins them completely. They just refuse to get creative at all. I often wonder how anyone gets any healthier eating hospital food. You can be certain that none of the quickly rising hospital costs are going to the kitchen. Why does it take years of study and great expense for medical people to realize what every thinking human being has known since the beginning of time? Fresh vegetables, fresh fruit and grains and a little bit of meat are what our bodies need. But that's an argument for another book. Here's a tip to the hospitals in America - don't overcook everything and add some flavor.

The next day they said I had to stay longer at the hospital and I said that I needed to get home. I made a deal that I would use oxygen if I felt like I needed it, even though I was no longer using it at the hospital since they got all the fluid off me, if they would just let me leave. They said okay and I left the following day.

Erin

By Sunday morning, he convinced the doctors that he was ready to go home. He was diagnosed with altitude sickness which, in his condition, became more severe than normal. But he was ready to be sprung and agreed to meet us at the Denver airport to fly back home. Sean and I arrived a couple hours before he did. I told him to call me as soon as he got to the airport so I could meet him the instant he got through security and help him carry his guitar.

I got back on the underground rail that takes you to the gates and rode it back to the security area. There's a long flight of steps that comes down from security. I stood near the train tracks and waited to see Pete come down the steps. Finally, after several minutes, I could see him with his guitar case on his back. He walked down the steps so slowly. As I started to walk toward him, he stopped at the bottom of the stairs, leaned against the wall and slid down till he was sitting on the ground. By the time I got to him, he was in tears and anxious.

Not sure what to do, I ran up to security and told them I urgently needed a wheelchair. Of course, they were not in as much of a hurry as I was, but eventually I got my hands on one while still trying to keep an eye on Pete at the bottom of the steps. I got back to him and helped him into the wheelchair. I think we both thought if he just didn't have to exert himself that he would be okay. But that wasn't the case.

I learned something that day that now seems so obvious. Even though an airplane cabin is pressurized, so you don't feel like you're at 35,000 feet, it isn't pressurized to be at sea level. Each airline is different, and you can actually call and find out. Southwest Airlines is pressurized at around 8,000 feet. I had gotten Pete to the gate where Sean was waiting and he was completely stressed out. He said "I can't get on that plane. I can't breathe."

I was completely unnerved in this new situation. We'd already checked all our baggage, including his meds (lesson learned that day), and we were already through security. As I pushed Pete in the airport wheelchair, we wound our way back through the airport and toward the exit. Along the way I was on the phone calling and reserving a rental car, one that we could do one-way. There was no shopping around for the best price. I just needed a car quickly.

Pete began to relax when he knew he wasn't going to have to get on the plane. I felt so bad leaving Sean yet again. She was 18 and well-traveled so I knew she would be fine getting back home with all our luggage and gear.

So back to the Weavers we went for the night. We ordered portable oxygen for our drive home from Denver to Nashville. It was a very peaceful evening after another nail biting day. The next day, we left early in the morning for Nashville. I did all the driving. Pete sat very quietly in the passenger seat. He was almost silent for two days of traveling. It was so unlike him.

We showed up in Dr. Fish's office the morning after we got home.

Pete

Dr. Fish informed us that he thought there may be a problem with the pacemaker/defibrillator he had installed approximately five weeks earlier. He had to go in again and redo the leads in my heart. I was not happy to hear this news. The last surgery took over four hours. This one would end up taking seven and a half.

Pete Huttlinger and Erin Morris Huttlinger

Chapter Four

The Stroke

I could have been planning a funeral
Picking out urns
And beautiful places to spread those ashes
Who to notify
Who to pay tribute

I could have been building ramps
New ways to enter our old life
Making new paths through our old rooms
Places for wheelchairs
Handicapped vans
I could have been buying stacks of notepads

So he could communicate with me
Writing with his good hand
Cryptic messages
Back and forth

I could have been interviewing nurses
Personalities that mesh
To help get through the day
To help him with everything
To help me with him

I could have been explaining to the kids
How their stepdad has changed
How everything will change
But how we will endure
And love him exactly the same

But I'm not.

I didn't have to plan, build, buy, interview or explain
I didn't have to weep for years
I didn't have to endure a new way of life
Or see all our dreams crushed
Or lose the music
He survived the stroke
He walks. He speaks.
He plays his guitar
He plays his guitar
He makes the most beautiful sounds
And they fill every corner of this house
Every corner of my life

– Erin Huttlinger

Erin

So, after all the mental preparation for heart failure… Pete had a stroke. A massive stroke.

It was Wednesday, November 3, 2010. My son James and I were just 10 minutes away from walking out the door for school. I was in the kitchen packing lunch and I heard Pete coughing. It was a harsh cough. Because of the heart issues, Pete coughed a lot, but this was different. I was concerned that maybe he needed a drink of water, so I opened the bedroom door. He was rolling back and forth on the bed and it wasn't a cough at all. He was trying to talk. But he couldn't. I thought he was having a nightmare so I threw the light on and told him to wake up, that he was having a bad dream. His eyes were wide open and panicked looking and the right side of his face was sagging. He was making noise but no words were coming out. I knew instantly that he was having a stroke. I could not believe it. Even as I was problem-solving in my mind, I thought to myself, "Are you kidding? A stroke? This is not at all what we've been preparing for."

I told him to stop trying to get out of bed, to lie still. He wouldn't — or couldn't— listen. I ran to the phone and told him not to move. I dialed 9-1-1 as I was running back to the bedroom and trying to hold him down with one arm. After I gave the operator all the details I hung up. I begged Pete to stop trying to get up but he was so confused and couldn't figure out why half of him was paralyzed. Next I ran to the other side of the house to find James. "James, we've got an emergency." He was very calm and I told him to run outside and flag down the ambulance. Then back to Pete. By then he had succeeded in falling out of bed. My poor sweet Pete was sitting on the floor beside the bed and looking so sad and confused. He finally gave up trying to move so I tipped him over onto his side and got a pillow for his head. I kissed him and told him everything was going to be okay.

The paramedics arrived and started asking me so many questions, and I was grabbing wallets and insurance cards and all the things you really don't ever want to have to think of in a crisis. Thankfully I was able to lay my hands on everything quickly. I was so stunned I couldn't even decide whether to put clothes on. I was still in my pajamas. But I pictured myself in the hospital in my nightgown and decided it was best to dress.

About that same time they were rolling Pete out of the house toward the back of the ambulance. I must have looked panicky because the EMT told me not to worry, that they would wait for me. I assumed I could ride in the back, but that wasn't the case. I had to ride up front with the driver. I just wanted to be in the back with Pete. I wanted to hold his hand and tell him not to worry. I was so afraid that he was frightened back there.

In the past, Pete has had heart surgeries and hospital stays. I always worry but generally I don't like people to sit and wait with me because it almost makes me worry more. But this was more than I could handle on my own. So I used the time in the front seat of the ambulance to start making calls. The first one was to Dr. Fish, as always. I live in fear of doctors who aren't tuned into Pete's congenital issues, doing something that will hurt him. A lot of his vital signs don't match that of a normal person. If misinterpreted it could lead to huge problems. So I left an urgent message for Dr. Fish. I was afraid to call my parents because it wasn't even 7 a.m. yet, and I didn't want to startle them too much. So I called my business partner and friend Alison Auerbach. I told her what was going on and that I needed her to meet me in the ER at Vanderbilt Hospital. My next call was to my brother Jason Morris.

I asked him to meet me as well. They both arrived quickly.

As soon as we arrived Pete was rushed into a trauma room. There was a team of neurologists and nurses that pounced on him. There were also two physicians from Dr. Fish's cardiology team. They were asking him a lot of questions which, of course, he could not answer. One key question that we were asked over and over and over again was, when was the last time he had been okay? All I knew was that I had seen him when he came to bed at midnight and he was fine at that point. By now that had been over seven hours ago. Time is crucial when it comes to treatment of a stroke. I knew that in the back of my mind, but I was treating it kind of like it was just the standard line of questioning, such as age, medical history, medications. But all of a sudden the light bulb went off over my head and I realized they were trying to determine what they could do for him, if anything. Even though Pete couldn't speak, I knew he was aware to some degree. And it hit me. Pete was on a lot of diuretics for his heart failure. He was up and down several times a night to go to the bathroom, and every morning he would recite those times to me when I'd ask how he slept the night before. He'd say, "Well, I slept okay but I was up at two and six." So, I told the doctors to ask him. I said he always knows what time of night he gets up to go to the bathroom. So they asked Pete in their loud voices, trying to shout through whatever fog he might be in. "Mr. Huttlinger, when did you last get up to go to the bathroom?" Pete held up four fingers. Jackpot! The winning answer. Four o'clock in the morning was the last time he knew that he was okay. It had only been about three and a half hours since he was normal. There were options. There was some hope that he wouldn't remain paralyzed and speechless the rest of his life.

A beautiful, older petite woman stuck to me like glue. She was assigned to the family members of those in trauma. She rubbed my back and informed me as to what was going on and what the next steps would be. Something of a tour guide for those unaccustomed to the intensity of a trauma ER. At one point she sat me down and told me that there was going to be a flurry of activity and a lot of doctors in the room with Pete. She didn't want that to cause me anxiety. I gently told her that if I didn't see a flurry of activity and a lot of doctors THEN I was going to be anxious. I wanted to see things happening and quickly.

They started to roll Pete out of the room. My tour guide informed me that they were taking him for an MRI. "Stop! I cried." "He can't have an MRI; he has a pacemaker/defibrillator implanted." They looked surprised. I can only hope that if I hadn't been there to tell them that that they would have discovered it on their own when they took his shirt off and saw the scars on his chest. An MRI machine is such a large magnet that it could have killed him to have it done with a metal device in his body. So they determined that they'd have to give him a CT scan. It wouldn't be as accurate, but might tell them what they needed to know.

I sat in the empty room by myself for just a moment. Then one of the cardiologists returned and sat with me. He wasn't one that I knew but had on his best bedside manner and let me know that it was too soon to know how he would fare but that there was no reason not to be optimistic. Just then my "escort" returned, and Alison and Jason rushed in. They looked as scared as I did. There were a lot of hugs and then we all divided up who needed to be called – my parents, my sister, Pete's siblings.

As Pete was being rolled back into ER from his CT scan I was finally able to go over and hug him and kiss his cheeks. He looks so baffled and he tried with every bit of strength he had to say something to me. As I leaned over him I put my ear close to his lips as if to hear him better. But it didn't matter because he couldn't speak. He would drop his head back down on the table, so exasperated, but then try again less than a minute later. I tried to make him smile by putting words into his mouth. "I know what you're trying to say to me Pete. You're trying to say you love me." Of course he was probably trying to say a million different things, but I'm pretty sure he almost laughed because he knew I was teasing him. I was absolutely terrified, but the one thing Pete and I live by is the thought that laughter is the ultimate healer. It wasn't going to cure him, but it might give both of us a sliver of a moment of calm.

I was asked to step out for a minute while they put a catheter in for him. As I leaned against the wall I overheard one of the doctors going over the CT scan results. She wasn't aware that I was Pete's wife and looked very nervous. Obviously it wasn't good news. Instead of ignoring the fact that I had overheard her concerns, she invited me around the counter to take a look at the pictures. Alison was beside me. I have no idea how to read a CT scan, but it's obviously an outline of Pete's brain and there was a huge section, maybe 20% that was lit up in glowing red. The doctor informed me that that was the area of the brain that had been damaged by stroke. At that point I nearly fainted. I felt light headed and thought to myself, "This is it, I'm going to pass out." But I didn't. It's not like I already wasn't aware that Pete's condition was bad. He was paralyzed on one side and couldn't speak, but this picture of his brain made it even more horrifying. Dead? Part of his brain had been damaged and could be dead. I don't know if that's what they actually said or if it's just what I heard.

Right about that time I was called back into the room with Pete. I got as close to him as I could. I held on to his left arm and kept talking to him and kissing him with smiles. I couldn't imagine the panic that could have been going through him. Everyone was talking to him and over him, but he could not respond to anything. My patient escort stood and rubbed my back the entire time I was in there. She was so loving, but I was so stressed that it verged on distracting me. I said nothing because I appreciated what she was offering.

I was briefly introduced to the neurology team at this point. Dr. Riebau, Dr. Ayad, Dr. Velez, Dr. Ferluga. Then, thankfully, Dr. Fish walked in. A brilliant man, a good friend and just at the right time. He stood at the foot of Pete's bed. Dr. Markham, another of Pete's cardiologists, was also in the room. Dr. Ayad proceeded to tell me the situation. Pete had had a "major stroke." A large part of his brain had been cut off from receiving blood and had caused him to be paralyzed on his right side and had caused him to lose his speech. It was severe. There were two options. The first was surgery which would be "high risk." Dr. Ayad mentioned "high risk" several times. Option two would be to give Pete medications and try to treat the stroke that way. Based on my understanding of the options, I thought it would be best to treat him with medicine than a risky surgery where he could die. But I wasn't understanding fully the underlying message of what Dr. Ayad was telling me. Dr. Fish did.

He proceeded to give a speech to all the doctors and nurses in the room that day, which to my recollection numbered over ten. His comments began with "This guy is a world-class guitarist!" Keep in mind, when I arrived with the ambulance, I didn't run into the ER saying, "Save my husband, he's famous and the best darn guitarist you'll ever hear." I just asked them to save my husband. But you could see the surprise on the other physicians when Dr. Fish said this. He continued, "Playing guitar is a huge part of Pete's life and his living. I'm a musician too, and nowhere near the player he is. If I couldn't play music, I would be devastated. I know Pete well enough to know that he wouldn't have the quality of life he wants if he couldn't play." Then he turned to me. "Erin, if they don't do this surgery, Pete will never play again. You need to take the risk and have the surgery." I was stunned. First of all doctors rarely tell you what to do. They give you all the data and then kind of drop it in your lap. Not this time. Dr. Fish made it clear that the option I thought Dr. Ayad was giving me wasn't an option at all. The choice was to risk the surgery and possibly improve his situation, or don't do surgery and he would live, but not improve from how he was now. I had no idea that was the choice I'd been given. Thank goodness Dr. Fish was there and able to interpret the choices for me. I have no doubt I would have chosen the non-surgery option. But when he said I needed to take the risk, I looked at Dr. Ayad and said, "Let's do the surgery" and Pete gave a very shaky thumbs up. Our entire future, good and bad, changed at that very instant and I will never be able to express my gratitude to Dr. Fish as deeply as I feel it.

Within minutes Pete was rushed off to surgery. I kissed him again and told him I loved him and that I'd see him when he was out. The patient escort showed us up to the waiting room. By then my parents had joined our entourage as had James and my sister Rachel Serrato, who worked at Vanderbilt. Pete's sister T and cousin Cath Strong were respectively in cars and on planes by this point and headed to Nashville. And my poor Sean was in school in Liverpool, England. After high school she had auditioned and been accepted into the prestigious Liverpool Institute for Performing Arts, a school whose co-founder is Sir Paul Mc-Cartney. I couldn't bring myself to call her. I didn't know yet what to tell her. Pete had had a stroke and would be fine. No, I couldn't tell her that. Pete had had a stroke and might die. No, I couldn't tell her that. I really wanted to wait until he was out of surgery to get my bearings and then call her.

At that point I texted our coffee club (a regular group of about 10 of us that meet every morning at the local Bruegger's Bagel shop) and asked Alison to call Pete's best friend Steve Emley. In what seemed like just moments, a number of them were in the waiting room with me – Steve, along with Dave Sanders and Michael Campbell from the coffee club. This was a completely different scenario from my previous times in the hospital with Pete when I preferred solitary waiting. I was terrified. In my normal optimism, I felt confident that Pete would survive, but I didn't feel confident as to what condition he would be in.

Everyone around me was worried, but talking and trying to keep me distracted. I could barely converse. I didn't want to break my concentration in any way because I was concentrating on Pete being alright. They just kept talking and I kept nodding but not really listening. Everyone looked so worried. Nobody was able to say that he would be fine.

The beautiful new waiting room where we were seated was on the sixth floor of the hospital and had a glass ceiling. So all day long we could hear Vanderbilt's life flight helicopter take off and land, take off and land. And even in my state of terror I could still think how everyone that landed on the roof of the hospital could easily be in worse condition than Pete was. I felt so bad for them and their families.

Pete's surgery involved a "wire" being inserted into an artery through his groin. The surgeons had to thread this wire up through his body, around his inverted, deformed heart, up through his neck and into his brain—into the exact spot where a clot had blocked off blood to his brain. They then had to break up the clot without underdoing it, and especially without overdoing it and perhaps causing even more bleeding.

After nearly two hours Dr. Ayad came through the glass doors into the waiting room. He had to walk a long way around the couches and chairs to get to where we were all sitting in a circle. He didn't smile. It seemed to take forever. He sat down to talk to us all. I was sure it was bad news. It wasn't. He said that the surgery had gone well. That they had broken up the clot and that blood was flowing again. But he also said that they had no way of knowing how much damage was done and that they'd have to wait another 30 minutes and do another CT scan. At that point they could see if any of the brain tissue had come back to life. He said he'd be back as soon as he knew something.

This time when Dr. Ayad walked back into the waiting room, instead of making me wait until he sat down, he looked at all of us, smiled and gave a thumbs up. I remember it like it was yesterday. I didn't even know what it meant exactly. I just knew that the doctor who hadn't smiled even once that day, and who was very grim as to Pete's options, looked incredibly relieved.

Again he came and sat with us and said that the portion of Pete's brain that was injured now looked greatly improved on the CT scan. He said that they would keep him on a ventilator for a day, and keep him sedated, but when he woke up we would know more as to his outlook.

Dr. Ayad walked away and I finally cried. I had no control

over it. I was so relieved. Overwhelmed. Everyone put their
hands on my back to comfort me as I bent over my knees and
just shook with tears.

We were all so relieved. I was just waiting for the okay to go
into his room in intensive care, to see him. He wouldn't know I was
there, but I would know that he was there. When I was escorted
into his room it was pretty daunting. But I knew he was alive and at
that point, that was what I needed to know. He was on a sedative
that kept him asleep, but that they could turn it down every so
often and speak to him. He would respond as well as he could. So I
told him how well the surgery had gone and that he would be fine.
He didn't react, but maybe he could hear me so I kept talking hoping he would relax and feel assured that he'd be okay.

Once every hour, the nurse was to go through a ritualistic
checklist. They would ask him questions to see if he was able to
answer. He was moving his lips! He was trying to speak. It was
miraculous. I knew that I'd be able to hear his voice again, sometime soon. It was a great sign that the surgery had worked to
some extent. But none of his limbs on his right side were working still. "Mr. Huttlinger, move your left foot." It would twitch.
"Mr. Huttlinger, move your right foot." Nothing. "Move your left
hand." It would twitch. "Move your right hand." Nothing. This
went on for hours, through the night. Then late into the first
night after the surgery the doctor came in. He pulled the covers
off of his left hand and asked him to move it. With Pete's eyes
still closed, he would follow the instructions and he moved his
left hand. The doctor pulled the sheet back over his left side.
Then he pulled the sheet off of his right hand and instructed him
to move his right hand. Nothing happened. The doctor spoke
loudly again, "Mr. Huttlinger move your right hand." Nothing. So

the doctor covered his right side with the sheet again. Then I saw it. The sheet moved. It was a delayed reaction, but he moved his right hand. I stopped the doctor before he could leave. "He's moving it," I said. Sure enough it twitched again. And then his right foot. It was a huge event. The doctor was thrilled as were the nurses on hand. He was moving and his speech was coming back. A huge weight was lifted. There was hope that he could return to normal although at that point nobody knew what that would entail. But it could happen.

Over the course of the next few days, Pete was slowly taken off the ventilator. The cardiologists pushed to keep his blood pressure down because of his heart issues. The neurologists pushed to keep it up to make sure his brain received enough blood. Too much or too little could prove catastrophic. But I was so impressed with how all the physicians worked in Pete's best interest. There was no competition. It was medicine at its best. Everyone's expertise was allowed to shine through.

All the doctors were so thrilled at the success of the surgery that they videotaped him doing various tasks to show how all his limbs were working and to demonstrate his speech. Of course by now, everyone knew he was a famous guitarist so they wanted to see him play guitar. I kept interrupting that thought pattern and distracting the doctors from asking about it. And family and friends pushed in the same direction. Everyone wanted to see if he could play. But I didn't have to see a guitar in his hands to know that he couldn't play. He could barely feed himself. After a few days I kept getting pushed to bring his guitar into the room. I did, but I hid it in the bathroom shower stall so Pete couldn't see it. I knew it could be devastating to him if he'd lost his ability to play. And although I knew it was possible that he could eventually play, I knew that he couldn't at that point. Finally, after a lot of pushing even Pete became interested. He asked for his guitar and I had to admit to him that it was in the room if he wanted it.

So I pulled it out of the case. Pete's sister T and her husband Tom Vigour were in the room with us. Pete was sitting in a chair, which in itself was a huge event. Then he tried to play. It was a disaster. He could barely strum the instrument. And when he tried to play anything even mildly intricate, his fingers didn't respond. Tears were just pouring out of his eyes. Exactly what I had been trying to avoid. Tom pulled a handkerchief out of his pocked and leaned down to be at eye level with Pete. He wiped his tears away. It was the most touching thing I'd ever seen. Pete tried to play for another five minutes. Nurses were oooing and ahhhing over him, but they had no idea how he normally played so they didn't realize that it was a loss. Finally Pete asked me to take the guitar away. It sat there for another day before he tried again.

Over the course of the next five days, Pete's recovery was so miraculous that more than one doctor left our room with tears of joy in his eyes. Pete was released after seven days, and two days later was asked to come and speak at a stroke symposium Vanderbilt was hosting. This was nine days after a massive stroke. Yet again Pete became a poster child for medical research. But absolutely all in our favor.

Pete

I woke up after having a stroke. I don't know if I'd been asleep for minutes or hours but I was uncomfortable and I wanted to move. But I couldn't. Not at all. I was perplexed.

Did I know that my face was drooping?

No.

Was I aware that I couldn't speak?

Not in the least.

How did I feel about being completely paralyzed on the entire right side of my body?

What's the right side of a body?

What's a body?

I was confused to say the least. I remember waking up and groaning in bed. I remember Erin coming into the room and telling me to try not to move. Help was on the way. I remember that I needed to use the bathroom. I was on diuretics for my heart and I was up several times each night. I would recite the times that I got up to Erin each morning.

When Erin left the room, I somehow managed to get out of bed and I peed on the floor. The only thought on my mind was to get out of the bed. It must have been quite a sight to see. Me flopping around in bed with only my left arm and left leg working. Erin was trying to calm me down but I just couldn't understand what was going on. I didn't know that I had had a stroke. And being a little bull-headed it probably wouldn't have mattered if I had been able to wrap my mind around it. I wanted out of that bed. I had to pee!

The next thing I remember was being put in the ambulance. There were three men putting me in. I remember one of them was very overweight. He had a huge belly hanging over me. I remember thinking how bad I felt for him and at the same time hoping he didn't have a heart attack and fall on me. In spite of my situation, I was genuinely concerned for him.

Then we were at the hospital. A lot of commotion. Nurses. Doctors. Erin. Dr. Fish and Dr. Markham were there. More confusion. I had no idea of what was happening around me nor how long it was all taking.

Dr. Fish asked me a "yes" or "no" question. I tried to answer but I was unable to form the word. I had the answer in my mind but I couldn't get it to come out of my mouth. Frustration in my mind. Confusion. He put his hands on my feet and said something to me. I assume it was encouraging.

They were trying to figure out how long it had been since the last time I got up from bed to use the bathroom. That would give them a better time line on when the stroke actually occurred. I couldn't tell them. But then they finally came to me and asked the question. The one question that could solve the mystery. "Mr. Huttlinger, when was the last time you were up last night?" I held up four fingers on my left hand. The only hand that was working. I had gotten up at 4 a.m. to pee. Someone said something encouraging to me again and then I heard them say that they were going to do the surgery.

I woke up. I don't know if it was the same day or the next. Erin, my love and my rock, was there. My cousin Cath was there. My sister, T, was there with her husband Tom. I knew that this was serious. I fell asleep.

Memories are strange. I can remember something that I am so certain happened in the way I remember it happening and Erin can remember it happening in an entirely different way. I usually give in to her memory. Mine is not so good. I often times joke in my shows if I forget a lyric, or if I flub a lick on guitar, or if I get lost in a story that I am telling, that I had a stroke. The audience has a good laugh. But in fact I did have a stroke. I don't know what effect it has had on me long term. It is a great fallback though. "Honey, I'm sorry, I forgot to take the trash out. I had a stroke."

I recall various things about the week after the stroke. The worst is when Erin gave me my guitar. Erin, Tom and T were in the room with me. I was sitting in a chair and I tried to play. "While My Guitar Gently Weeps" is a tune that I like to play in my shows. There was nothing gentle about what was happening. It was a full on blubber-fest. I was sitting there sobbing as I tried to play and my right hand just refused to obey any commands. The most touching moment between Tom and me happened then. I was there crying. Trying to play. Tom, who was a forester complete with barrel chest and big moustache, grabbed his handkerchief and wiped my eyes. Then he wiped his. Then he wiped mine and his again. I was a fairly decent guitar player up to that point in my life. I had accomplished a lot but at this moment I was not a player any more.

There were several good things that happened in the week following my stroke. Bob Burwell came by to visit me. He took one look at the room and said, "Lighting. You need better lighting. I'll be back." A couple of hours later he returned from Target and had a floor lamp and two desk lamps. Plugged them in and my room was transformed from a stale hospital room to a place that was cool enough for a musician to hang out in. Thank God!

Dr. Nyad came by the room one evening to check on me. He was in his scrubs and he had his motorcycle helmet in his hand. He was ready to go home. I was sitting up in bed, trying to play something on my guitar that I shouldn't have been able to play. I had been trying to play each day and some of the basics were coming back to me. He flipped. He grabbed his iPhone and yelled for someone to come in and show him how to film with the phone. He wanted to document me playing but he didn't know how. He was quite literally a brain surgeon and couldn't run an iPhone. I laughed. Eventually he got it working. He was frankly amazed that I could move or speak at all, let alone get any sounds out of my guitar. He teared up before he left the room.

I had a lot of visitors over the course of the week. My old pal, Cynthia Manning Martinez, came by to visit me with her mom. She brought Ben & Jerry's ice cream, fresh salmon with green beans and she used just enough salt. Hospital food is just devoid of flavor but a little salt is okay. She wanted me to play my guitar for her to sing in my hospital room. She is a wonderful singer. I think I tried to play but it was not good.

Fellow musician and friend Jeff Taylor came by. He said we had a gig coming up in a couple of weeks and I needed to be there. It was at the historic Ryman Auditorium in Nashville. Man, is Jeff brave. (I ended up doing the gig. It, too, was not good from my perspective. But what a healing moment it was! On that show Aubrey Haynie, the most amazing fiddler I've ever worked with, told me not to worry too much. He said I might not be the same player I was and that maybe I'd just be a different player. I love optimism! That was all I needed to hear.)

Erin's friend and business partner, Alison Auerbach, decided I needed a massage so she bought me a two-hour massage to be done in my hospital room. I put a sign on the door when the massage began saying, "Please do not interrupt. Massage in progress." One of my doctors came by shortly after the woman began and he was not too pleased. I saw the humor in this.

I was released after a week. Then one week and two days after I suffered a "major" stroke I was back at Vanderbilt to perform for a Stroke Symposium that was being held there. I thought to myself what any musician would think – "free lunch." But the doctors thought something else entirely. I was a phenom. I had not only survived the stroke but I had regained almost everything I had lost. I could walk again, though my right leg often dragged and I could talk again. I could almost feed myself with my right hand again. I could play a tune on the guitar and that was why I was there. To play. So after a long introduction by Dr. Riebau where he showed detailed photos of my brain and talked extensively about my condition, I walked up on the stage, grabbed my guitar and played the one tune that I could get through on that day – McGuire's Landing. After I performed I fielded a few questions. One doctor asked me, "How many years has it been since your stroke?" "Years?" I replied. "It's been nine days!" There was a gasp followed by applause which I'm sure was for the doctors because I had done nothing to deserve it. They did the work. They saved me. All I did was show up.

When I walked off the stage and out of the room, I saw one of my surgeons, Dr. Velez, standing there with tears streaming down his face. I walked up to him to find out what was going on. He told me that this is not normally the way things happen after someone has a stroke. I was touched to say the least. I put my hand on his shoulder and said something encouraging to him. I felt so bad that he was upset and the gravity of the situation was not lost on me. I realized that I was one of the lucky ones to have survived.

However, my journey to becoming a guitar player again was just beginning.

Two weeks after I had the stroke I was sitting out on our back deck at home. Guitar in hand I was struggling to play something. Anything. As usual my left hand worked fine and my right hand just wouldn't cooperate. I was strumming some chords and our friend John Oates, of the Rock & Roll Hall Of

Fame duo Hall & Oates, and his drummer Jon Michel showed up. I remember thinking how nice it was that they would come over to my house to check on me. John heard me playing and said, "What do you mean you can't play? You sound fine. Wanna' come and do some gigs with me?" I replied the only way I knew how. I said, "Yes, if you're crazy enough to hire a guy who just had a stroke, then I'm crazy enough to accept." I had two months before the gigs and so I had a goal. Something to work towards.

After a little more time had passed, my friend Cynthia came over one day. She had a plan. She was going to come over every Sunday and sing and I would play. We've known each other since she was just 15 and I was just 16 years old. She is a great singer and it sounded like it might be just what I needed so I agreed. She suffered through my playing every Sunday for months on end.

"Damn it!" Erin would hear me yelling out from the sun-room where I often practice.

Cynthia also made me work on my ability to write. I couldn't write anything legible after the stroke. So one day Cynthia said, "We need a set list." So I sat there waiting for her to write one out. She started to and then she stopped and said, "I have an idea Pete, why don't you write one out for us? That way you can practice your writing and your guitar playing." Grrrr... She bought a notebook for me to use to practice writing.

The journey was truly just beginning.

Chapter Five

The Beginning
Of The End

Pete

I think I'd been getting sick for a lot longer than I was willing to admit at the time. Looking back from today's healthier perspective I can see the denial I was in. Erin would ask how I was feeling and I would usually say, "Like a million bucks." I was so used to saying that that it never occurred to me to say anything different.

When it became obvious how sick I was getting I can remember Ed, Erin's dad, asking with his beautiful, soft West Virginia accent, "How are you doing, Pete?" And I would reply, "Like a million pesos, which is about two hundred and forty bucks!" I remember being sick and looking up the equivalent of a million pesos in US dollars for the joke. Always the joke. The joke is so important to me. I believe that is a big part of my success in health and in business. Maybe not the joke itself but the attitude that accompanies the joke. Light hearted and carefree, I try not to take myself too seriously. I've worked for and with enough people who take themselves way too seriously in my mind and they don't seem to be happy to me. I would take happiness over any other alternative. Money. Sex. Drugs. Rock and roll. If those things made me truly happy then I would choose them. But they don't and they never have.

I would say I began getting sick in 2001, approximately 10 years before I suffered from end-stage heart failure (ESHF). My first wife and I were not getting along very well and that weighed heavily on me. I think that took its toll on my heart. Not that staying together would have prolonged my heart's integrity any longer.

I had stopped going to the gym for the most part a year before ESHF hit me. Though I do recall the last time I went to the gym. It was about a month before I went into the hospital. I told Erin that I just really needed a workout to blowout whatever it was that was making me feel so bad. I got to the gym and started with the treadmill. I like treadmills because with all the read-outs they have (heart rate, calorie counter, speed, incline) they are a good gauge of my fitness. I climbed on and I couldn't have walked more than a minute - slowly - and I stopped. Trying to catch a breath that was proving elusive. I started again and walked about another 20-30 seconds and stopped. I told Erin I was done for the day. I was genuinely worried at that point. I knew my heart was getting sicker and there was nothing I could do about it. I had to fight a little bit of depression around this time. I'm sure it was just the helplessness that I felt and feeling trapped inside a sick body.

Erin

After Pete had recovered about 70% from his stroke, we decided it was time to go out on the road again, to begin touring. We wanted to start slowly so we did one solo show in Connecticut and it was wonderful. It was at a small venue and the promoter there was willing to book us knowing that Pete might not be recovered enough to play when it came time for the show. But he could play, very well in fact. The audience was thrilled to be a part of his return to health. They were supportive and Pete just came to life being on stage again. It took so much work to get his unique skills back, but he did it and it paid off. The next weekend we did a show with John Denver tribute artist Jim Curry. Pete was a "side man" which means he was a performer as part of someone else's band. This is a little bit less pressure because he wouldn't have to carry the entire performance. I did notice that he became very tired during this weekend of shows. It was so hard to tell if it was his heart giving him trouble and slowing him down, or if he was still weak as he recovered from the stroke. He was improving and declining at the same time so we were fooled as to his health status in many ways. But I knew he was having to really struggle because I drove most of the way from show to show that weekend, and carried the suitcases and guitars. I know that is not Pete's preference. It makes him feel uncomfortable to have to relinquish those things to me. But he also is acutely aware of his limitations—and as painful as it is to him emotionally, he knows when to give in and just allow me to be the roadie.

He slept a lot on that trip. And he walked more slowly. And he coughed a lot. We had no idea that his heart failure was about to kick into full gear. But it did. Within days after we returned from that trip Pete was in the hospital. He was having great difficulty breathing.

One sign of heart failure is the ongoing battle with fluid build-up in the body. Even though Pete began taking diuretics several years earlier, he continued to battle fluid in his lungs. So we spent almost a week at Vanderbilt hospital in mid-March. And we thought he was doing so well. He had intensive IV diuretics, for days and days. He couldn't sleep lying down. He couldn't sleep sitting up. He was beginning to have anxiety attacks. As I look back I see now that he was drowning in a way. But after days of treatment, they sent him home.

For the rest of March and April he alternated being in the hospital for a week and home for a week. I think perhaps the doctors knew the situation was getting worse and perhaps wanted him to be able to spend more time at home. But Pete and I are practical and frankly felt safer in the hospital than we did at home.

Over these next few weeks he went from walking slowly, to walking with a cane, to walking incredibly slowly with a cane to not being able to get off the couch. A 49-year-old active guy brought to a screeching halt.

Pete

Our friends Kevin and Pat brought over a walker for me to use. I had already been using a cane sometimes. They knew I felt bad using a walker but they said that if I needed it I should use it. That made perfect sense to me. Kevin is a 9th degree black belt in martial arts. He had presented me with an honorary black belt after I survived the stroke, and now I had a walker. I told them I did not deserve a black belt— they assured me that I did. The cane I had already been using I had received as payment for some music I helped Kevin with for an instructional video for one of his martial arts teachers. His teacher made canes used for fighting but, luckily, they were just as functional for a sick guy who needed a hand.

Erin

Pete began suffering from panic attacks and could not sleep at all. Not only was he taking handfuls of pills, but he also was on an IV of Milranone that was carried in a bag over his shoulder and dripped through a pump and into a PICC (peripherally inserted central catheter) line. Pete has no recollection of this time period. He knows he was terribly ill, but he has been able to block out a lot of the anxiety and hospital visits.

When the anxiety attacks started to happen I knew he needed some anxiety medication. I'm not a doctor, but I could see the panic in his eyes. He couldn't breathe, he couldn't sleep and possibly in the back of his mind he knew his body was dying. Pete saw his mother die from emphysema and he watched her slowly lose her ability to breathe deep breaths. It was horrible for him, and now he was experiencing the same crisis, but for different reasons. I was able to get a prescription for Xanex, but it didn't help with the anxiety and just put him in a constant fog. He hated it.

As we were going through these weeks of demise, picture this: Pete is just like the child he probably was in the hospital following his first operation at age 12. He's the kid that you see in the movie that everyone loves. As an adult, in great pain and underlying fear, he still gets to know every single nurse and doctor on a personal level. Just like he's meeting fans after a show. He asks them questions about themselves, and then follows up with them days later. "How was the marathon you ran?" "How did your daughter do on the test?" "Did you get any sleep after your last shift?" He cares so much about people that while he was dying he would wonder how they were doing. He would ask them questions, and joke and flirt. Nurses, doctors, administration. They were all going to connect with Pete whether that was their original intention or not. Some walked into his hospital room prepared to make a quick getaway. But once Pete engaged them, they often sat and talked for quite a while. He would have the sourest of nurses giggling before they left his room. It is really an amazing thing to watch.

Meanwhile, when I say we went to the hospital, I really mean we. I lived, worked, ate and slept in the room with him. Not only was it imperative to be there early enough to catch the doctors doing rounds, but I knew that he felt better with me there. And with shift changes every 10-12 hours, it was really crucial to be there for some sort of consistency. Pete couldn't always do it for himself. Everyone in the hospital needs someone close to their side to take in the tons of data that are available. We were fortunate enough to be in the care of major medical centers, but even then the patients need someone to speak on their behalf when they just don't have the energy to do it for themselves.

I always left the house with my laptop, a bag of clothes, books, a pile of work, all sorts of chargers for phones, computers, etc… and on more than one occasion a bottle of wine for late in the night when Pete was sleeping and I couldn't. I would curl up in the cozy yet uncomfortable pull out couches and chairs in various hospital rooms. I would watch TV late into the night. My one moment of peace each day. I would talk to Sean and James who were at home. I would wander to the all-night cafeterias for snacks to have with my glass of wine. Eventually I would stop worrying and drift off to sleep until Pete called for me or when the doctors would wander in doing their rounds. During the night I would think of questions to ask the next day, and write them down in my notebook. A notebook I still carry with me. As soon as the doctors would throw on the lights and come in, often before 8 a.m., I would be dressed and ready with my notebook of questions. And they always answered them in as much detail as I wanted and never made light of any of my concerns. I will always appreciate them for that.

Chapter Six

The Trauma

Erin

With Pete's health obviously in a rapid decline, we were coping but confused. Weeks on and off in the hospital, caused high anxiety in all of us. As optimistic as Pete is, he never waived me off and said he was fine. He never told me to go home to sleep. I think he knew I needed to be there, for comfort, for safety.

In mid-April it was made very clear to us that Pete needed a heart transplant. Instead of "managing" his heart failure, everyone shifted quickly into heart transplant mode. I was surprised at how relieved we were about this. It was almost exciting. Pete would get a transplant, recover, and our life would get back to normal with Pete feeling better than he had his entire life. We were made aware of the issues that go along with transplants, but it didn't matter. He was virtually incapacitated as it was, so anything would be an improvement. So our spirits were lifted. We were fast-tracked to getting a transplant.

There are three levels on the heart transplant list—The United Network for Organ Sharing. Pete was going to rocket to the top level because of the severity of his heart failure and the fact that time was running out. Within days of being readmitted to the hospital we met with numerous social workers, we met with administrative people who were working with our insurance company, and we met with drug specialists who talked to us about medicines following the surgery. Pete was put through a battery of tests to make sure that he had no other health issues that would make him less of a candidate for transplant. It was all terrifying but exciting at the same time. Pete passed all the tests with flying colors….except one. He was very healthy, with the obvious exception of his heart, he was cancer free, he was young and active, he was emotionally healthy and was able to work and offer something to society. But he had abnormally high lung pressures, known as pulmonary hypertension. If Pete received a healthy heart, it would fail once it was implanted because of these freakish pressure readings. Everything came to a grinding halt. Everyone was scratching their heads—which happens a lot with Pete.

So, the new problem of the day was how to get Pete's lung pressures down. One approach is to put a patient on Viagra. Ironic isn't it? All dressed up and no place to go, so to speak. In fact Pete was put on that "little blue pill" three times a day. They also put him on tons of diuretics. And then checked him again. Nothing. No reaction to the treatments. His lung pressures were still extremely high.

Pete

Heart Transplant. We had been concentrating on nothing else. Get my lung pressures down and get on the list. Lung pressure is so important to heart transplant patients because it is an essential part of the heart's working environment. In my case, because my heart's ventricles are reversed, it's like there is a clamp on the blood vessels going into my lungs. So when you install a heart with normal pressure coming out of it, the blood will blow back out of the lungs and into the new heart. The lungs can't handle normal pressure and the new heart can't handle the blowback from the lungs. The result is that your body ruins the new heart. It's an awfully tricky situation.

But getting your lung pressures to go down is not like studying for a test. There is nothing you can actually do to improve your odds. You can't sit in your chair and take five really deep breaths every minute and then check it and see that they are down. You can't run up a hill and make them go down. You can't change your diet and have them magically lowered because it's not like cholesterol. You can't do the "wait and see" method to see if the pressure will lower on its own. It takes medicine and a lot of luck. I had plenty of the former and I was running out of the latter.

Dawn Eck is a nurse practitioner and was our point person at Vanderbilt when we started the heart transplant process. She was wonderful in working with us to make sure that we were a good family who could handle the stress of a transplant patient. That we were financially stable. (We weren't rich by any means but we were okay with our money.) And that emotionally we were ready for this big leap. We were and she was convinced of it.

We saw Dawn almost daily and she always spent time with us when she came in the room. She didn't just give us the facts and leave like doctors do. She seemed genuinely interested in us as people and that was a nice change of pace at a hospital.

Erin

All the fuss, all the commotion preparing us to be rushed into surgery when a heart is ready came to a screeching halt. We noticed that nobody was coming into the room any longer. Just the normal rounds. The social workers disappeared. The nurse practitioners disappeared. The administrative folks stopped asking us to sign papers. It was just too quiet. We knew something had changed. The doctors even started looking at us differently. It was tremendously disconcerting.

We continued to ask what the next steps would be and all of a sudden we were getting very vague answers. Finally, Pete just put his foot down and insisted on knowing what was going on.

Pete

Sean and Erin were there with me. I was lying in the bed and they were sitting in chairs in the room. We were just talking quietly about something inconsequential when Dawn showed up. Dr. Leniman was with her. The air changed when they entered the room. It was heavier. They closed the door behind them and both of them had very forlorn looks on their faces. They explained to us that a decision had been made that I would not be put on the heart transplant list. My lung pressures were just too high to risk losing a good heart on me. I couldn't believe it. I had been their star patient for 12 years. Always working out whenever I could. Eating well. I always watched my weight. What did they mean, I couldn't get a heart? We were dumbfounded.

Erin, Sean and I teared up after they left the room. I had been given a death sentence with no appeals. We packed and headed for home.

Erin

Home again, with an IV pump and a ton of new medicines to take. Lots of logs to keep measuring Pete's weight, his input, his output, his blood pressure, his temperature. Anything we could monitor from home. We were signed up for home health care and were treated royally by Sandy, our visiting nurse. She later told us that she had never treated anyone that was so sick, yet still at home. She admitted that she was terribly worried Pete would not survive.

Our last week at home was horrendous. Pete remembers none of it. He doesn't recall Sandy, or the IV pump, or the fact that his sister came for a visit. He was so miserable that he couldn't sleep or eat. Of course, I know now that his heart had enlarged to the point that it almost filled up his entire ribcage. It was so huge that it could just barely pump. Pete didn't play his guitar for weeks and that is the ultimate sign to me that he was dying. Nothing could keep Pete away from his beloved guitar. Until now. He used a cane to walk from our living room to the kitchen. He would sit at the dining room table and try so hard to eat, but everything came up within minutes. He was withering away. His heart was so ineffective that his stomach couldn't get any blood to digest food. So it was rejected. I can only imagine the level of exhaustion he must have felt. He hadn't slept for weeks, couldn't get a deep breath and wasn't able to get any nourishment. I get tired just writing about it.

We asked Kevin and Pat to pick up an old recliner from my mother's home and deliver it to our house. I rearranged the bedroom to put the chair in there thinking that at the very least we could sleep in the same room. Me in the bed and Pete in the recliner, because for the last month we had alternated, one of us on the couch and one of us in the bedroom. Just so he could get some rest. Nothing worked. He was deliriously tired.

Yet, every couple of days we would trek into the hospital for blood work. It took every ounce of energy he had just to get out of the car and into the elevator.

The kids were worried. They would come by the hospital room after James got out of school, and sometimes join me in the cafeteria for dinner. I was always very specific and up front with Pete's condition. I could be because I had no idea the trauma that lay ahead. They are smart kids and seemed to process all the medical information very well. Sean was always full of questions and would subtly try to figure out what the future held. She was so grateful to be back from school in Liverpool, where she had been when Pete had the stroke. She couldn't have been any more grateful than I was. She took over the mother role with her brother on those days I was with Pete. I felt like I stayed very optimistic for both of them, but they know me well enough to know that things were not going well.

Near the end of April he had his final blood work done. I got a call that night from Connie Lewis, one of our wonderfully supportive nurse practitioners. She had grown very close to us over the last few months. She asked if Pete was with me, and I said that he wasn't. She said, "Erin, Pete is a very sick man." Now this is something, of course, I already knew, but when she said it out loud it took on a whole new meaning. She wanted me to read between the lines. She told me that he needed to be in the hospital and quickly. Up until then we had kind of insisted upon being admitted. This time they were insisting. She told me to take the evening and to get things together and to get him there the next morning. I could tell by the firm way she was talking to me that his situation was getting very dire. Why they don't actually say it, I'm not sure, but I think in a way I'm glad they don't. It might be too much to cope with. Or maybe they knew me well enough that I just need to know what I was supposed to do, and I'd do it.

And it worked. I came home and started getting our bags packed for another stay at the hospital. I did whatever I could do to help Pete sleep but it was impossible. I didn't matter if he sat up or stood up. There was no position that tolerated the fluid building up in his lungs. He absolutely couldn't get any sleep. Which, of course meant that I didn't get much either.

This would be our last stay at Vanderbilt for quite a long time.

When Pete arrived at the hospital this time, the tone was quite a bit different. All of a sudden all the doctors were much more serious and they looked so much more baffled. And I noticed that they weren't talking to me as much, weren't keeping me as filled in. They were desperately trying to get Pete's lung pressures down so he could get the transplant. But nothing was working. And Pete and I were living every minute to hear the results of each test for lung pressures. We really believed that they were going to say, "Okay, it worked and now you are on the official transplant list." Those words never came. Each time we'd get the results was another huge disappointment. We kind of knew we might be running out of options, but we also never, ever gave up and we knew the doctors weren't going to give up. It's my sense that even though Pete's congenital heart defect has caused him major problems in his life; it has also gotten him some of the best treatment in the world, due in part to the fact that it's such a rare condition that he becomes a "study." So more doctors get involved in the case. There are so many unique abnormalities that it takes more specialists and I believe that has worked to his advantage.

The doctors decided to put a balloon pump in one of Pete's main arteries. It was a last ditch effort to get his lung pressures down and also to get some blood circulating in his body. Pete was hurried off to have the procedure done. All of his main physicians stood around and talked to him before he went in. I kissed him before they rolled him out. Although every time they take him away from me I am nervous, I had become pretty used to these types of procedures where they go through his neck or groin to get to arteries. I wasn't worried. But Dr. Fish was there, too, and he suggested we go have coffee. That frightened me. He's a busy man and was, I'm sure, juggling more patients than just Pete that day. We walked down the hall to Vanderbilt Hospital's massive cafeteria and both grabbed something to drink. Dr. Fish always looks serious when he has his physician's "hat" on, but this time the look was deeper than serious, it was worried. We talked for about half an hour and he prepared me for what was likely to happen. He told me that when Pete's gets out of the procedure I am most likely going to be told that he has to go to another hospital. Most likely it would be Texas Heart Institute (THI) in Houston. That Vanderbilt would transport him and he would receive an LVAD (Left Ventricular Assist Device). In Pete's case it would actually be an RVAD (Right Ventricular Assist Device) since his ventricles were opposite the norm. Generally these are referred to as VADs. A ventricular assist device is a mechanical pump that's used to support heart function and blood flow in people who have weakened hearts. The device takes blood from a lower chamber of the heart and helps pump it to the body and vital organs. These devices in their portable form have not been around very long at all. They had been available but the patient would be plugged into a huge device that would mean they couldn't leave the hospital as long as they were on this pump. But now they are portable and ground-breaking. Dr. Fish explained the numerous reasons why Vanderbilt could not implant Pete with the device and why Pete would be in good hands in Texas. He told me to be ready for this news and he told me that I need to be prepared to stay there for "a while." I am forever grateful for this bit of "head's up." It gave me time to process it before Pete would hear it. I could be strong for him in case he was frightened.

The reality of all this was finally starting to make my head spin. This was really snowballing in a way I never imagined. I hadn't even recovered emotionally from the stroke. But I knew what I had to do and as long as I have in my mind that there is something that needs to be done in order to move forward, I can keep from breaking down. So I just kept trying to solve the problem. As long as there are options, I can stay positive. As far as I knew, there were still options. I still had a while to wait before Pete would get out. So I raced back up to his hospital room and started packing our things. In my over preparedness for these hospital sleepovers, I always had extra clothes, my laptop, a huge file folder with work, phone chargers, iPad, etc... The one thing we didn't have was any legal documentation. No Medical Power of Attorney and no Will. I rang up a good friend that lives outside of Denver, Colorado. He was a friend through music and a lawyer. Many times he had told me that if we ever needed anything that he could help us with, to please ask. Now was that time. I called his cell and gave him a brief synopsis of our situation. As with most of our friends, he already knew Pete was sick, just not how severe it had gotten. He certainly could hear the panic in my voice even though my words were stable. He dropped everything he was doing and wrote up a Will for Pete. I couldn't stand to even think of needing it, but Pete and I have a very strong and practical side, and I knew if he were able to think clearly, he would have told me to do it. Within an hour I had an email and had it printed. I slipped it into my briefcase for Pete to sign later.

When Pete came out of the procedure, he was awake, but in no condition to discuss a will. Dr. DiSalvo and Dr. Lenneman told us exactly what Dr. Fish predicted they would. That Pete couldn't wait to get on the transplant list and that he needed to get an LVAD, and quickly. His organs were failing – his liver and his kidneys were failing. If we OK'd it they'd be on the phone making final arrangements with THI and they would engage Vanderbilt's LifeFlight (a King Air B200 fixed wing aircraft with two pilots and two flight nurses.) Of course we OK'd it.

Pete was hurried off to Intensive Care. At that point we started seeing teams of doctors preparing him for Life Flight. Kidney doctors, liver doctors, cardiologists. We would be leaving in a matter of hours. Since the balloon pump was in the artery in Pete's groin, he had to lie perfectly still and flat. It was not long before his body started to feel a lot of pain from being so rigid. Even with morphine, he moaned all through the night. I would get out of my sleeping chair in the hospital room and go over to massage his back and help relieve some of the pain. I had watched the nurses do it earlier that evening. They would slip their hands under his sheets, then under his back and then draw their fingers across his back over and over again. He was so appreciative.

As soon as we got to Intensive Care I put the call into our close family and friends and told them what was happening. Both Sean and James hurried to the hospital as did my mother. Pete's best friend and our best man, Steve also came to see him before we left. It's the first time I saw the kids really scared. James, who is comfortable in almost any situation, had difficulty standing by the bed and talking to Pete. For the first time he really looked like someone who was seriously ill. The tons of diuretics flowing through his system were making the weight drop off of him almost before our eyes. We had no idea how much of his body was actually fluid that he was retaining. Since his heart could barely pump, the fluid built up in his tissue. But now he was getting thinner by the minute, like a balloon losing its air. So James sat in the chair by the window and when his sister and I urged him to come over and talk to Pete, he couldn't do it. He was visibly shaken. Sean was, too, but she knew in her heart that she might not see him again so she made herself talk to him and smile and hold his hand. He was dopey because of the morphine, but also because his body was slowly fading on him.

I tried to keep my smile on and even though I didn't try to pretend like everything was okay, I always let them believe that everything would be okay. And in all honesty, I truly did believe it. I just didn't know when everything would be okay.

The preparations were coming at me at rapid speed. All the doctors came to give me information. The nurses were changing shifts. I was talking to Pete and trying to make him smile and be encouraging. And then Dr. Fish called with some fantastic news. He was given the green light to fly with Pete to Houston and also fill in the doctors on that end, in person. Yet again, I was overwhelmed with relief and gratitude. I know that face to face communication is always best. And even though they had supplied us with an 8 inch stack of papers and numerous DVDs with Pete's entire medical history encased in them, nothing could replace Pete's friend and long-time doctor arriving in person, at his side. His appearance would speak volumes. It would let Texas Heart Institute know that this was an important guy and that they were being trusted to save his life and that we were ALL counting on them. Including Dr. Fish. Not many doctors make the flight with their patient. So I thank him and I thank Vanderbilt for approving it.

So Dr. Fish and I filled out all the necessary paperwork to be allowed on to life flight. Our bags were very limited as it was a small plane.

Around 7:30 the next morning we received word that the plane had landed from wherever it's previous run had been, and that within a couple of hours they would be at the hospital to get all of us. We would be transported by ambulance from the hospital to the small John C. Tune airport in Nashville. The flight nurses, who arrived with their special (very small) gurney, were amazing guys — as positive as you would ever want to meet. They knew exactly what they were doing. But we were blind-sided by one thing. They said that if both Dr. Fish and I went that they would have to stop and re-fuel along the way. They were willing to do it, but I was not. I convinced Dr. Fish that it was far more important for him to stay at Pete's side than it was for me. I could hold his hand, but Dr. Fish could save his life. I knew he knew I was right although he looked like he felt bad leaving me behind. I quickly booked myself a Southwest flight from Nashville to Houston and I would arrive only two hours behind them.

Pete was very aware of what was going on, but now remembers very little of it. Moving him from his Intensive Care bed to the flight gurney was a huge undertaking. There were so many wires and monitors. The balloon pump had its own unit the size of a microwave that kept the blood flowing. He had catheters sticking out of both sides of his neck. IVs were in both arms. He had bottles of medicines and fluids going into the IVs. All these things had to systematically be disconnected and reconnected to the portable units. Finally he was lifted carefully onto the gurney. They tightly wrapped a sheet around him, much like a newborn infant, then buckled the belts over him in three places to keep him secured. The only thing showing was his face, and he was still able to smile. I kissed him over and over again and followed the flight nurses and Dr. Fish down the elevators, through the Emergency Rooms and out to the ambulance that was waiting to take them to the airport. I kissed him once more and told him I'd see him in Houston. Then I gave Dr. Fish a hug. How could I not. Everything was in his hands at that point.

The ambulance pulled away and there I stood. I didn't have anything to do at that point. Nothing to keep me running and on high alert. I just had to wait 'til I could go to the airport and catch my flight. Unfortunately, it was too early in the day to have a glass of wine, but frankly my days and nights were so turned around I almost could have. But I haven't found a hospital yet that had a bar in it.

I figured it would be a long time before I would be able to

eat so I stumbled to a nearby restaurant. Half tired and half ready to faint. I was definitely alone. Pete and I are such a close couple that even when he was at death's door, I still felt like we were a team. Even when he couldn't speak to me, I never felt like I was alone. Because we were locked together in so many ways, that I just need to be in the same room with him to know everything would be okay. It's only when he was out of my sight that I felt lost.

Sean came to get me and took me to the airport. She's a strong kid. Lots of worry, but lots of optimism. A lot like me. I am proud of the way both the kids handle trauma. They had certainly seen a lot of it over the past year.

She dropped me off at the Nashville airport. I had a suitcase that my brother had dropped off at the hospital for me the night before. I haphazardly threw everything I had in the suitcase — clothes, books and papers. And I had my backpack with laptop, purse and credit cards. I knew all I needed was something clean to wear on any given day and my work. Nothing fancy, no makeup, nothing.

I always wondered how people could show up to work after a death in the family, or if they had a really sick child. My first encounter with this was when I was in my early 20s. I worked for RCA records. A woman named Donna worked in the accounting department there. Her brother passed away, and the next week, there she was, at her desk. I was dumbfounded but couldn't ask her about it. How can you come back to work the week after your brother dies? How do you ever come back to work after something like? But I think I understand now. By this time, work is engrained into your system. It's what you do every day. It makes everything normal. And I had to work. Pete and I are both self-employed, he as an entertainer and me with my publicity and artist management company. And without Pete working, I really had to hang on to every client I had. Fortunately I had two amazing partners…my mother was one and Alison Auerbach was the other. We all shared clients and the two of them backed me up. Normally, if something was going on, I could work from anywhere and frankly nobody knew. I could be in my office in Nashville, at a private show in Alaska, or even on vacation. Most clients never knew the difference. But the difference this time was that I was too mentally fractured to work. I could do general housekeeping type assignments, but that was it. I had always been very anxious about letting my clients know, ever, that I wasn't available to them 24/7. Entertainment PR is such that you never know when a client might be in need, and it certainly isn't limited to eight hours a day. But this time was different. I couldn't juggle. I needed to be 100% in the present moment with Pete.

So the night before we left Nashville, I wrote to everyone and let them know my situation. Every single client I had was very supportive and concerned. I guess it's good karma after 30 years of being in this business. Thank goodness. It was such a gift from all of them to know that I had a small window in which to breathe and try and get beyond this crisis – even though I had no idea how long it would last.

When I arrived at the airport, I was still light-headed and somber. I had been through that airport a thousand times. But for the last eight years, it had almost always been with Pete. So I was missing the other half of myself. It was a terribly strange feeling. But I didn't feel panicked. It was almost like it was out of my hands for a few hours and I had no option but to relax, give into it and be present. So after I got through security I wandered around and found my gate. I still had over an hour. So I went to one of the massage kiosks they had. I think it was $35 for 30 minutes. I wished the masseuse good luck and told her if she could get my neck and shoulders to relax that she deserved an award. It really helped and stabilized me. I paid the money, lined up and boarded the flight. A sweet woman next to me offered one of her free drink tickets and we both ordered a glass of wine. Then I closed my eyes.

Pete

I can't stand whiners, complainers and the like. Merely sitting on your butt and complaining does nothing to alleviate a situation. There's no problem solving involved. No action. Unless you are planning on using the complaints to achieve some goal, stop it. What possible good can ever come from grumbling, nitpicking and moaning? I have very little respect for people who can do but choose not to. Whiners.

I remember when I was checked in to the Texas Heart Institute at St. Luke's Episcopal Hospital. There was not much going on and they had my bed, with me strapped to it, sitting in a hallway. I thought they were going to rush me off to surgery as soon as I arrived. Turned out that there had been a little miscommunication between Vanderbilt and THI. THI thought I was coming in the night before and had given away my room at the hospital. Dr. Fish had a few words with them and they were working hard to get a room for me.

They got one and then it started. A nurse came in and saw my 'picc' line. That is a permanent IV line usually placed in the inside of your upper arm or sometimes in your leg. A deep vein is accessed this way and the patient can go home and avoid the need

70

for IV's to be changed every three to four days. It's like your own little port where you can give blood and get meds all from the same "One-Stop Shopping" store. She said something rather unflattering about the people at Vanderbilt who put it in. I stayed quiet though I wanted to jump from the table and defend the folks who'd been working around the clock to keep me alive. A little while later, she said to herself, but loud enough for everyone in the room to hear, and she was obviously agitated.

"Why in the world did they just do one line?"

A little while later there were two of them in the room and they were both complaining about my single picc line. I was getting tired of the complaining.

"Why would they just do one picc line?" the first one questioned.

"I guess they don't know what they're doing over there in Tennessee?" replied the second.

I couldn't take it any longer.

"Why in the hell don't you just rip it out and put it in the way you want it? Then you can stop all your whining," I said. I continued, "I've been pretty happy with the treatment I've received from Vanderbilt and I don't appreciate hearing you constantly putting them down. Maybe they do things differently but that doesn't make them wrong. They did what they needed to do to keep me alive."

My words fell on deaf ears. They didn't even acknowledge me. These nurses were not interested in hearing me going on about the accolades of Vanderbilt. They just wanted to have something to complain about. I guess nurses are just regular folks too.

The pain in my back was increasing from having to lie flat for so long. The morphine drip was running beautifully and so I recited the Serenity Prayer quietly to myself.

"God grant me the Serenity to accept the things I cannot change, Courage to change the things I can and Wisdom to know the difference."

At this point I could do nothing to change my situation and I was wise enough to know it. I needed no courage. I had morphine.

Erin

The minute I was able to get off the plane at Houston Hobby, I called Dr. Fish. He sounded elated and said that Pete was in good hands. I knew he had been worried about that. Dr. Roberta Bogaev was now in charge and he said they were medical "soul mates." Thank God! I was so happy to know that he could go back to Nashville feeling like they had made the right decision sending Pete to Houston.

Pete's sister T was driving from Mississippi, racing to get there because we thought he would be rushed into surgery for the heart pump. His brother Frank and his wife Wendy arrived from Los Angeles the night before and were there when Pete was admitted to Texas Heart Institute. And now I was on my way from the airport. Even though I "relaxed" somewhat on the flight, the minute I hit the ground in Houston I couldn't get to him fast enough. I know Pete feels better and reassured when he sees me and I was worried that he was looking for me.

It was a strange feeling arriving at Texas Heart Institute. I felt really angry. This wasn't home. Vanderbilt was home. I didn't know these halls or this cafeteria. The smells were different, the nurses and doctors were different. The procedures were different. The rooms weren't the same and they noticeably were missing chair/beds in the rooms. And wait a minute.....VISITING HOURS? Are they kidding? I am used to 24 hour access and I'm not leaving this man. I cried when they told me I wouldn't be able to spend the night. I thought they were cruel. I thought Pete would be scared if I left. I hadn't realized yet that he was so sick that he might not even know the difference whether I was there or not.

When I finally saw him and he mustered a smile, I was so relieved. He looked like he had lost 20 pounds overnight, and in fact he probably had. I was frightened because he was starting to look really old. He couldn't move much, and the parts he could move had stopped. He was holding himself so rigidly that he was holding his arms up across his chest with his hands kind of curled up under his chin. He stopped turning his head and would just move his eyes. He became more rigid with each passing day.

Eventually he stopped talking unless absolutely necessary. The doctors postponed surgery for a few days. In part, they still needed to get the lung pressures down or it wasn't a good idea to do surgery. The other reason was because they had to educate themselves. Pete's anatomy has baffled some of the best doctors in the world. And Dr. Bogaev was no different. Nor was Dr. Bud Frazier, a world renowned cardiac surgeon who was scheduled to do the surgery. They studied the huge stack of medical files that Vanderbilt had sent.

At the end of the first night in Houston, as I was, cruelly in my mind, told that visiting hours were over, I walked past Dr. Bogaev sitting outside of Pete's room. I mentioned to her that I had been told to be prepared for Pete to be in the hospital for a while.

And although I would never dare to rush her, could she enlighten me just a bit as to what "a while" might look like. She smiled as if she'd been asked this question many times, and said, "Let's just say that if you get out of here in three months it will be because everything is going absolutely perfectly, and that isn't usually the case." So, I went to the hotel and slept on that a while!

Over the course of the next several days many, many doctors came and went. I didn't get the same warm and fuzzy feel as I did from the docs at Vanderbilt. But I was very impressed by their matter of factness and their positive energy. It was obvious that even though they had never worked on someone with Pete's anatomy, they did work with some of the most challenging cases day in and day out.

So we were introduced to their team way of working at Texas Heart Institute. We met several people from the "liver team," and the "kidney team," "infectious disease team," "surgical team," "congenital cardiac team," etc… They came in one or two at a time. Every time a doctor would walk into the room, Pete's relatives and I would pop out of our chairs to hear what they had to say. They were always quite appropriate and would talk directly to Pete, who was flat on his back. But I would intercede, whether they liked it or not, and answer on his behalf and interpret for him. It was difficult for him to hear sometimes and very difficult for him to talk. He was being seriously dehydrated and had no moisture in his mouth. Besides, by that time he was starting to let his mind wander for self-preservation purposes. The doctors were all very responsive to me and always answered all my questions. They never seemed rushed, and generally made us feel like they did this type of surgery every day. But actually they didn't. They did heart pumps every day, but not on people with Pete's physiology.

As each day ticked by, Pete became less and less communicative. His hands drew up until he was holding them near his chin and he just moved his eyes. It was as if he thought he was paralyzed. And he became more and more dehydrated. As part of the prep for his surgery they needed to get all extra fluid off him and to get his lung pressures down. This involved his virtual dehydration.

The day he went into surgery he lightly grabbed my finger and put it in his mouth on his tongue. It felt like sandpaper—rough sandpaper. It was a shock. No wonder he didn't feel like talking to anyone. There wasn't an ounce of fluid left in his body. I was surprised that he wasn't a little pile of dust in the middle of a hospital bed.

Pete's brother Frank and sister T and Frank's wife Wendy were all so diligent. Rarely was Pete left alone. I'm sure it's possible at some points he wished he would have been left alone. But we were all so worried about him needing something and not being able to get what he needed. I was consumed by that but also worried that I would miss even one doctor coming in. I was an information sponge. I would soak up every single detail of Pete's diagnosis. Partly so I could understand, partly so I could relate it to others, and partly so I could cross reference all the other doctors that came in. It was baffling to me that they could keep track of all the information that was processed there, and I thought maybe I would be helpful in that way. And I was at times, but it turned out that their communication system at Texas Heart Institute was very meticulous and every doctor, generally, knew what had happened earlier in the day. Keep in mind that Pete was given medicines of some sort every hour or even constantly via intravenous drips. There were tests being run and blood being drawn constantly for days on end. So in my mind the data was overwhelming, but I did my best to keep up with it all. On top of that I was the one person that knew Pete intimately. I knew every twitch, every smile or lack thereof, I knew how to read between the lines of what he was saying. And virtually all of this knowledge I learned as his manager, not his wife. So, right or wrong, I felt that it was my responsibility to convey his thoughts. As if I was Annie Sullivan (Helen Keller's devoted teacher). I thought I was the one connection between Pete in his disconnected state, to the real world. If I wasn't there, then Pete would have no voice. I know that people survive without their soul mate to speak for them all the time. But why do it that way if you don't have to? I was there for a reason. I have to have a purpose or I would have just curled up into my shy self and felt helpless. I couldn't feel helpless.

After we were in Houston for two or three days, the doctors had had time to review the scores of medical records on Pete. It would make sense that it would take days because the amounts of information were massive. He had also had numerous tests. It was late one evening. Dr. Bogaev came by the room to give us some test results. At this point I can't even remember which test results it was. But as she was leaning over Pete's bedside and talking to him, she mentioned, very briefly… "Since you aren't transplantable….." blah, blah, blah… I didn't hear the rest of it. Something to do, I'm sure, about the LVAD device being the end point and no longer a "bridge to transplant."

I was absolutely stunned. Stopped dead in my tracks. Everything that we thought we had been working toward was just shot. Pete didn't flinch. He was so sick that I didn't even think he'd heard it let alone taken note of it. I was truly distraught and this was the first time that I didn't have my best friend to lament things with. I went back to the hotel room. T was already asleep. I had several glasses of wine and pondered what our future, if there was a future, would be like. It was one of those moments where the whole game changed, right when you thought you had the game plan figured out. I had to do some serious meditating on things to not get depressed. It was one of those windows where I had a conscious decision to make. Become overwhelmed, or keep moving forward and figure out how to solve the next on-coming problem. Although I wasn't happy, or even optimistic, I got through the night and tried to figure out how to discuss this with Pete.

There were signs all around the ICU floor that no flowers or fruit baskets were allowed. I'm not sure why but no doubt they had good reason. And I'm not much of a rule breaker; however, as I was walking to the hospital one morning I kept walking past beds and beds of marigolds. They were all around the medical center area. And they smelled so good. Pete's favorite flower is the marigold and each spring I would always plant some big pots around the outside of the house. So I picked one marigold and carefully put it in my backpack. When I got into Pete's room I waited until there weren't any nurses around. He had become completely rigid—not moving his head or arms or legs. Just look-ing straight at the ceiling. I pulled the tiny marigold from my bag and leaned over Pete. I told him I had something special for him and held the flower just under his nose. I told him to breathe in. He instantly recognized one of his favorite scents and smiled. Randomly throughout the days in the hospital I picked marigolds from the beds around the hospital until they didn't bloom anymore. I would slip them into his room and let him smell the outdoors. My intention was to relax him and to give him hope that he would be able to pick them for himself someday.

On Tuesday, after we'd been in Houston for five days, the doctors said that now was the time for surgery. Tomorrow was the day. I was relieved and terrified. I hate being in the waiting room. That is always my biggest fear. I am absolutely traumatized at the thought. But I know that people do it every day, so I steadied myself. T and I went back to the hotel and had a drink. Frank, who had had to go home to work for a couple of days, flew in and got to the hotel about 3 a.m. the morning before the surgery. He slept hard and fast. The three of us were back at the hospital by 6:30 in the morning.

The surgery was delayed a few hours. We were exhausted, but hopped up on adrenaline and caffeine. I so wanted it to be over for Pete's sake. I really thought it would be an instantaneous miracle cure. I look back and am surprised at how little I knew and now how much I've learned. Those hours of delay were difficult. Like ripping a band aide off slowly. It's less painful to just tear it off quickly. But just when we thought we'd be seeing him off to surgery it would be delayed.

Finally I escaped to get a diet soda (my sickening habit and caffeine source). Of course, as was always the case, if I left for a moment I'd miss something. The elusive Dr. Frazier came into the room to talk to Pete. Frank was texting me to get back to the room. I was racing there to catch Dr. Frazier and I encountered him in the hallway outside of Pete's room. I was relieved. Dr. Frazier told me that the FDA had approved a special dispensation (called "compassionate use") to allow Pete to get the HeartWare pump, which was technically still in clinical trials. Not only had he gotten that approval, but he also got approval from our insurance company, thanks in no small part to our insurance angel Elizabeth Talbot, to pay for a device that was not yet FDA approved. It just goes to show how much weight Dr. Frazier wielded. But after asking questions and getting all this information, I made the mistake of asking about Pete's likelihood of survival. I would hate to say that Dr. Frazier's bedside manner leaves something to be desired. Since this moment I've come to understand his methods a bit better, but at this point I was a wife who really needed the surgeon to tell her that her husband wasn't going to die on the operating table. Up to this point, as stressed as I was, I truly believed that everything would be okay even if it was scary. But when I asked Dr. Frazier if he thought the surgery would be successful he said that he couldn't make any promises and that "bleeding is always a concern." Then he patted my shoulder and walked off. I almost fainted in the hallway. All it would have taken was a "don't worry Mrs. Huttlinger," or maybe an "I've done a million of these and never lost anyone" type comment. But I didn't get that. So my world turned around yet again. It set the tone for the next excruciating nine hours.

Pete was prepped for surgery. As we knew they were going to roll him out of the room at any moment, Frank suggested we all hold hands and say a prayer. It was beautiful. It seemed like the right thing to do. And it helped all of us. But it made Pete that much more aware of how dire his situation was. It was enough having one of his brothers and his sister show up to be by his side and mine, but when Powers of Attorney were being signed, relatives flying in and prayers being said around you and over you, it was disconcerting and comforting at the same time.

I had the Will, but couldn't bring myself to have Pete sign it. I knew that it was the smart thing to do, but also, my concern was Pete and his fragile mental health in the midst of his extremely fragile physical health. How would he feel if I had him sign a Last Will and Testament on what might have been his deathbed? I decided it wasn't worth the risk to even have the slightest bit of doubt implanted into his mind. If I lost everything, I would have preferred that to thinking that I might have done something to make him doubt his only chance of survival. So I kept the Will hidden in my briefcase.

After the prayer a slew of nurses, doctors and aides came up to disconnect Pete from all his power plugs, pumps, and IVs. He looked so helpless. But he didn't look afraid. I think he was too sick, and in too much pain to even care. We were all in tears. We tried to keep it hidden but I was sure that he could see me crying and I was so scared that he would think he was dying based on my reactions.

With about seven people in tow, Pete was wheeled to the elevators. T, Frank and I rode down in opposite elevators. We reached the surgical floor at the same time and reached out to kiss Pete and tell him goodbye and I know in all of our hearts we were so worried that we really were telling him goodbye. I was heartbroken. We were then escorted to the "waiting" room. It should be called the "excruciating waiting" room.

As soon as we arrived in the waiting room we were met by a very kind volunteer. He helped us get checked in. We registered with the front desk and were told that every hour and a half, a nurse comes in and reports in to all the families. So T, Frank and I all found our comfy seats. Trying to pretend we felt normal when we didn't really feel normal. We tried to read books and magazines, but our minds were definitely wandering. T took time to call her husband Tom and her daughters, Frank or I would reach out to Colleen Solomon, Pete's first cousin who is the disseminator of all information to the Huttlinger clan. Colleen is special for orchestrating all things family related. She has an amazing email blast that she sends out with good news or bad news. Prayer lists. Graduations. Weddings and family adventures. Newborn photos. Colleen was born to be a cruise director, but she spends her time educating the nation through her work with Scholastic (one of the largest publishers of children's books.) Anyway, I digress. We all reached out with our phones to those that could spread the word as to the current status.

To the best of my recollection I didn't call anyone. I was in a semi state of paralysis. I texted the kids and my parents and those closest to us. The first report came in....Pete was prepared and they were beginning the surgery.

Frank looked very worried. We started talking. It took a lot of effort to even think a sentence through let alone convey it in spoken word. But we both did. I thought that maybe asking Frank about some funny stories Pete had told me, might make him laugh. He told me some funny times when they had gotten into various types of mischief. But then all of a sudden Frank teared up and said, "I should have been a better brother to Pete." It caught me off guard because Frank has always been a wonderful brother to Pete and I wanted him to know that Pete felt that way. So I reassured him. But that moment frightened me because it made it clear that Frank was not sure Pete would survive the surgery. Of course, how could he be? How could any of us be?

Several hours went by and each time the nurse came to check in with us, I was just relieved to know that he was still alive. I can't even remember what the updates were, but the fact that there even was something to update was really all I cared about.

In the background of this week, Frank and his wife Wendy had been working furiously to find a place where I could stay long-term. The hospital gave us several sheets worth of information and they ran down every lead in their spare moments. They had settled on an extended stay hotel that was within walking distance, since I didn't have a car in Houston. It also had room for relatives to stay as they came and went, and the crown jewel....a kitchen. Being vegetarian and health conscious I can only eat out so much.

Frank got a call that the room had opened up a day earlier than we expected. This would save us over a hundred dollars where we were currently staying. So, as soon as the reporting nurse gave us an update, we shot out of the hospital to switch hotels. We knew we had exactly ninety minutes before the next report. And not to mention the fact that it gave us something to do that was distracting and that we couldn't feel guilty about.

So we hustled to the car, drove to the hotel, packed furiously and checked into the new hotel. It was hard to get excited in the midst of this day, but I was excited about my new home away from home. I couldn't wait to get the refrigerator filled with healthy food. I had been living on Diet Coke and Kashi bars for weeks.

Even as I write this I feel the tension brewing in my body. The day was so anxiety ridden that I can't believe we all didn't end up in the hospital. In fact, I wonder if a study has ever been done of waiting room casualties. So, as the tension and stress was building and building and we were waiting to hear how Pete would do, I got a call from my daughter at home. "Mom, the guys are here cutting down the trees." Pete had orchestrated this be-

fore he ended up in the hospital. A couple of dead trees needed
to be taken down. "That's great Sean, thanks for letting me
know," I replied. "But Mom, are they supposed to cut down the
huge cedar tree in the backyard?" WHAT? I told her quickly, that
no they weren't supposed to and to stop them. But it was too late.
They had cut down the 60-foot centerpiece to our backyard. Who
would think that after all we had been through that this would be
the thing that would flip the switch on my stress levels. Sean is a
kid that is as sentimental as I am. Sentimental about almost everything that we come in contact with.

My head was spinning. I could have burst into tears. I was
tying everything together in my mind. The tree gone, is Pete
gone? Tree dying, Pete dying? Too much change. Too much
stress. I told Sean that I couldn't process all this, that Pete was in
surgery and I was afraid that I was just going to have a nervous
breakdown. So I hung up.

At that moment I realized that I do have control over one
thing. I have control over how I'm going to mentally process this
stress. I was at a precipice no doubt. I was just about ready to go
over the edge. But I knew that it would do nobody any good and
that it wouldn't even give me any relief. It would just give everyone else one more person to take care of.

Sean was stressing out as well, and I knew I had to call her
back so she'd know I was okay. But what would I say? I wanted to
scream. So I came to the decision that the situation with the tree
was a test of some sort. A test of how we would handle this. A
test of our ability to prioritize. A test of whether we believed
Pete would be okay. That's a lot of tests. I called her back. "Okay,
kiddo, I have caught my breath now. Here's what I think. I think
that this whole tree fiasco is a test. It is a test of our strength dur-

ing a very, very trying day—a trying year. I figure we can either let this issue put us into hysterics or, better yet, we can use it to show us what is really important today. And what is important is Pete. He's the one who needs our focus and our energy. We can either allow ourselves to be upset by our tree being dismembered, or we can realize where our priorities should be." Always in step with me, Sean immediately said, "Well, there is a lot more light in the living room now that the tree's out of the way."

That's my girl. And all the anxiety of the loss of the tree went away.

It was a huge turning point in my day, and hers, and a moment I have accessed many times since then. At the very most difficult times, there is still a moment when choices are made. There is always some control that can be exerted even when you think you have no control over anything.

My day wasn't over yet. I still had a husband in surgery, and I was still worried. But at that point I felt much more hopeful all of a sudden. The three of us rushed back to the waiting room. There was still nearly 20 minutes before the reporting nurse was scheduled to return. So I left T and Frank there and went to the cafeteria to get my thousandth diet Coke of the week. And, as was par for the course, Dr. Frazier came while I was gone. When I returned only minutes later Frank and T said that Pete was out of surgery, although they were still closing him up and finishing up certain things, that everything had gone well and that I was to call Dr. Frazier. I was given a number and dialed his office. He said that not only had Pete done well, but that the surgery had taken less time than they imagined it would. At least seven hours. But as was his usual manner, just about the time I was going to say "Yippeeee," he commented;

"Now we just have to hope that his kidneys wake up." Pete's kidneys were in shock from the balloon pump, the lack of blood flow and malnutrition. He said they often "wake up" after a few days, but not always. Damn. He certainly never let me get too excited for long. But I do appreciate his candor, because frankly it was a time for honesty.

Either way, I was relieved beyond description. The heart pump was in and was working very well according to most indicators. The true test remained to be seen.

I called Dr. Fish right away. He said he'd been waiting to hear from me and felt that he could breathe easier now. That said a lot, too. To know that he was unsure of the outcome made it clear that Pete had been, and still was in, a very tentative situation. Nothing about this surgery was routine.

We waited another hour and a half or so, and were then allowed to go in and see him. Cardiac post-op critical care is an amazing place. Even though I was on edge, I was no less amazed at the intensity of the care available there. I would venture to say that most, if not all, of the patients on that floor not only didn't know they were there, but to this day they probably have no recollection of it. It was like the patients were some form of alien life that had been captured and were on life support. The "rooms" were the size of horse stalls. In the middle of the room was a huge hospital bed. The bed took up about 80% of the room and was surrounded by every life support system imaginable.

The walls were filled from side to side and top to bottom with machines that were lit, and/or making noises. Lots of tubes and wires connected the machines to Pete. The machines seemed more alive than Pete did. They were making breathing noises and sounds of heartbeats. And at the foot of the bed was a small desk. At that desk sat a nurse inputting data by hand onto a massive spreadsheet. That nurse, sometimes female, sometimes male, was constantly glued to all the machines and constantly making notes. On this particular floor there were many patients. It was an amazing sight.

As we approached Pete's room, I became pretty uneasy. Dr. Fish had mentioned to me on the phone that sometimes after this type of surgery, the chest isn't closed right away. It's a safety precaution in case they would have to go back in in an emergency, say if there was internal bleeding. So he told me to be aware of that and not to be frightened. They would close his ribcage, but the incision might still be open and probably would be covered with a type of plastic. So I approached very tentatively.

I peered around the corner of the room so I could ease into the shock of what I would see. As it turned out he wasn't completely closed, but he was covered by sheets so I would never have seen anything. Thank goodness we knew he was okay because it sure doesn't appear that way at first. There were numerous large tubes coming out from under his sheets. Blood was coming from these tubes into a bag beside his bed. These apparently were chest drainage tubes and were letting all the fluids caused by the surgery drain out of his chest cavity. There were a lot of loud monitors. He had catheters sticking out of both sides of his neck. And he was on a ventilator—a huge tube that went down his throat into his lungs and breathed for him. He looked asleep and relaxed. There were no signs of pain on his face. And there beside him on the bed was a nylon bag that looked a lot like a large camera bag. It contained a controller and two large batteries. Out of the bag came a wire that ran straight into his abdomen. It was the wire that was attached to his heart pump. This four-pound bag was now a permanent appendage.

I thought that he must be on the verge of dying. How could anyone look like that and be anywhere near good shape. But the nurses were so encouraging. They smiled and told me how great he was doing. "Really?" I was shocked. They seemed totally comfortable with his situation and seemed happy to answer my many, many questions. They understood that we were nervous and explained all the machines and monitors. By the time we left I was a brand new person. I gave Pete many kisses that he'll never remember. But he looked so fragile that I didn't try to hug him or squeeze his hand. There were too many IVs in his hands and arms to even try. It was more likely that I would hurt him than help him.

Since our phones didn't work in most of the hospital, the three of us hurried out to the lobby where we had clear signals. Each one of us went to different spots and started making calls. I think that I called or texted every single person that I knew, or that knew Pete. Since we'd put the word out on Facebook and via CaringBridge, many, many people around the world were on pins and needles. The relief on T and Frank's faces was encouraging to me as well. We were all smiling and even laughing, the relief was so intense.

It was a wonderful day. A huge hurdle had been jumped. I don't really know what I expected beyond that day, but I really thought that the hard part for Pete was all behind him. That now he would recover just like people do from any surgery. After most open heart surgeries the doctors have you up and walking the next day and out of the hospital in four or five. I thought that he had gone to the brink and didn't fall off, so we just had to get him up and active and we'd be outta' there. I was so incredibly wrong. We remained in Houston nearly four more months.

Chapter Seven

Sean & James

Erin

During this time period, my kids, Sean and James, were 18 and 16 years old respectively. Up until the February before Pete's heart failure, Sean had been in Liverpool, England in college. I was disappointed when she said that the program at LIPA wasn't right for her and that she wanted to come back to Nashville, but it was the best thing that could have happened. She knew that she was devastated when Pete had the stroke and she was out of the country.

It was so stressful for her to be so far away. She felt helpless.

But because of her decision, she was on hand when all hell broke loose. She is a huge crutch for me and seems to have inherited those of my traits that are the best. It is my understanding, from her younger brother James that if I am not around, she more than sufficiently fills my shoes. I don't know that he particularly likes it, and I don't know that she likes it. But Pete and I both love it. She becomes the mom figure as if she has been brain-washed with my thought processes.

And James is a willing participant. At just over 6' tall, and built like a linebacker, James could be a tough kid to handle. But he's not. He's gentle and supportive and even though he doesn't often verbalize how much he worries and cares, it's obvious he does.

During the brunt of Pete's heart failure, the kids had to take care of themselves in a lot of ways. Even though I tried to stay on top of the deadlines, appointments, money, etc….They had to take care of everything else including our dog Denver. And it was a lot. The kids and I had worked really well as a team, especially since we had all been through divorce together. Now I wasn't carrying my weight for them, but there was nothing I could do.

Pete says that all that was a great time of learning and self-reliance in their lives. And I think he's right. I don't think I was ever left a night alone in my life until I moved out of the house after high school. These kids were left at home for four months.

And I can't slight my parents in any way here. They were the back up for everything. They were the safety net and the love and support system in my absence. My father spent the night many, many nights so the kids would feel safe. My mother stepped in with pet sitting for our dog Denver whenever necessary. My brother and sister were there if the kids needed anything, including food, and they made sure the kids were kept involved in any family celebrations. Mom and Dad attended school events in our absence. But mostly they tried their best to keep everything as normal as possible. I've heard that discussed when very young kids are involved in a tough situation at home. Family members try to keep their schedules and daily life as normal as possible if their parents are out of the picture. But I've learned that it is just as important for older children. Their lives had been turned upside down. They were in fear of their step-father dying and I know that they were equally worried about me and how I was holding up. I would speak to Sean every day from Houston, sometimes several times a day. James is less fond of talking on the phone, but I would call him or text him, nonetheless. Even if he didn't feel like filling me in on his day, he still knew I was interested and just wanted to hear his voice.

Over the course of our time in Houston, from late April until late August of 2011, James finished his sophomore year and began his junior year in high school. He got through exams and all the details and excitement of putting another year behind him, but he did it without any of his parents around. His father lives in Pennsylvania and Pete and I were obviously out of the picture. But James' demeanor amazes me. He is so strong and so steady. He handles all adversity well. I do believe that he is stressed by some things, but I also believe that he has tapped into a very mentally healthy place so that he can deal with each day as it comes. He doesn't worry in advance and he doesn't lament the past. It's very unusual for such a young person to feel that way. The whole family tries to emulate that trait in James.

When August rolled around, and we were still not home, he

had to head off to marching band camp and get himself registered for school, again with very little help from me. And since he
didn't yet have his driver's license, he arranged transportation for
himself to every stop on his busy schedule. He never even trou-
bled me with it.

I bred into Sean all my anxieties. She is a clone of me in many
ways. And then she has a whole set of anxieties on her own. But
it makes her an amazing kid, a great songwriter and singer, and
hopefully a stupendous mom. It also makes her a great person to
leave in charge. She worries about the house, the dog, and most
importantly, her brother. I didn't want her to be stressed, and I
spent a lot of my time away talking her out of being anxiety ridden and sometimes it was more than I was able to take. But in the
end I knew I was better equipped to handle stress, so I took on
her problems too. On those days, my father was really the one
who would talk her off the ledge. Ironically since Sean is such a
mirror image of me, my father can talk to her in the same loving,
humorous, logical way that he did to me back when I was in high
school....and college.....and later in life. The same techniques
worked for both of us. So thank goodness for him, because I
think that sometimes you just need someone other than your
mom, or dad, or stepdad to offer guidance.

Two teenagers left alone, for an entire summer, with money
and a car, a hot tub and a big house, normally would be recipe for
disaster. But Sean and James didn't take advantage of their situation. I believe that they are cautious kids and I believe that they
knew I couldn't handle one more problem.

Chapter Eight

Tragedy Averted

Erin

Once Pete survived his surgery, there was so much unknown territory in front of us. I took a deep breath, and again, we moved forward. As fast as everything had deteriorated over the past month, I had no idea that the recovery wouldn't be nearly as rapid.

Pete's favorite guitar is a Collings OM-1 cutaway –He calls it "God's Guitar." Collings is owned by Bill Collings, and Steve Mc-Creary heads up the Austin-based company. Both have been incredibly supportive of Pete's career in many ways and we've grown close over the years. On the Friday morning following Pete's surgery Steve called me from Austin to say he wanted to fly in to be with us. I told him that Pete was unconscious and wouldn't even know he was there. He said that it was okay. He wanted to just see him and to sit with me for a while. It was so kind and I welcomed the visit. I assumed that Pete wouldn't have wanted many people to see him in the situation he was in. It was scary and unnerving for the observer. But I knew that Pete loved Steve and that he would have approved the visit. Steve showed up at Texas Heart Institute right about visiting hour. So I took him up to the post op ICU. I cautioned him, but he wasn't deterred. He stood by Pete's bed, patted his head gently and talked to him for about five minutes. I could see that it took Steve's breath away to see his good friend in that condition. After that we headed to the cafeteria where we sat and talked for a couple of hours. I wasn't shaking in my boots anymore so I was able to be still and just enjoy the conversation and support that Steve offered.

Pete remained in post-op cardiac intensive care for five days. They kept him on the ventilator for three of those days, until they were able to take him back into surgery and close his chest. Once that was done, they slowly weaned him off the ventilator. It wasn't any easy transition back to breathing on his own. Apparently Pete must have liked the ventilator doing all the work because it was nearly 24 hours before his lungs started to do a portion of the breathing on their own. Then a little bit at a time they took over and he started to breathe without the ventilator. He was never without additional oxygen, but he got off the ventilator. Then things started to improve. Once the breathing tube was out, the nurses could turn off the meds that kept him asleep all the time. Gradually he woke up. Four days after the surgery he opened his eyes. By this point T had had to return home. So Pete awoke to see me and Frank.

The visiting hours were extremely limited. We could see Pete only four times a day for 30 minutes. 5:00 a.m., 10:00 a.m., 5:00 p.m. and 8:00 p.m. Frank and I would wake up at 4:30 a.m. and hustle over to the hospital just to spend a few minutes with Pete. Sometimes he was awake and sometimes he wasn't. The nurses were always working intently on him and happy to give us a full and detailed report. After all this time in hospitals, we usually had a pretty hefty list of questions. The best part is that Pete would know we were there. He didn't smile but he could respond to questions with short answers. His voice was just a whisper. Between the ventilator tube and being dehydrated for weeks on end, his vocal chords just didn't work very well.

Frank and I took every opportunity possible to visit Pete. We often didn't stay the entire 30 minutes because it seemed tiring to him. Or maybe it was just tiring to us. It was not the type of room with a chair, or anywhere to sit. In fact there were so many cables and machines and lines going into and out of Pete that I was always worried I'd trip over something and "unplug" him. Pete and I grew up in the era of great cartoons like Bugs Bunny and Road Runner and of great comedic TV shows like Carol Burnett and The Lucy Show. So we relate a lot of things to comedic, cartoon situations. So as I tiptoed around his bed and feared tripping over something vital I knew that if Pete were himself, we would be joking about accidentally tripping over his life support systems and all the comedic opportunity that would offer.

That Sunday Frank headed back to Orange County. He was really wonderful about juggling his work and visiting Pete. It was the first time since arriving in Houston that I was alone with Pete. It was very quiet but I could be extra attentive to him and in the time away from the hospital I could be attentive to myself.

Pete was coherent enough to know that he was okay but it became obvious that he was forgetting certain things and maybe couldn't remember exactly that he was in Houston or how he'd gotten there. The nurses told me that it is common because it's so difficult to get any rest in a hospital, or to know if it's day or night. So one morning, as I walked to visit him I brought my iPad and took pictures all along the way—photos of the hotel front, the skyline of the medical center, flowers, and the entrance to the Texas Heart Institute. Pete was slipping further and further into what they called ICU psychosis. He was saying things that made no sense at all and was speaking less and less. So I showed him the photos and explained where he was. He said he knew that he was in Texas but couldn't get any more specific than that. Then I showed him pictures of the outdoors and explained when it was daytime. I also asked the nurses to please put on time appropriate shows…The Today Show in the morning, Oprah in the afternoon, then NBC Nightly News (our favorite) and later in the evening the late night talk shows. Anything to help him get his bearings. It didn't seem to help. There were no windows and no way to differentiate day from night. The lights in ICU were on brightly 24 hours a day.

After several days, he was not any more aware of what was going on, but they had him sitting up in his bed. I was pleased to see him upright. It was the first time he hadn't been flat on his back in over two weeks. I'm sure it felt good to him as well. Soon we were moved to Cooley 8A—Cardiac Intensive Care, and named after Dr. Denton Cooley, the founder of Texas Heart Institute and famous for the first implantation of a total artificial heart. We would stay here for nearly three weeks.

Pete lived in his ICU psychosis for over a week. I was told it would likely last a day or two. But he was just as distant and incommunicative the next day and the next. It began with him just saying things that didn't make sense. He would talk about seeing things that weren't there. But eventually he just started talking less and less and less. He stopped responding to the doctors when they would come in. They would ask him if he knew where he was, why he was there, what his name was. But he would say nothing. I just couldn't bear it. So one day I put my face close to his face and held his hands tightly. I asked him what his name was. He just gave me a silly smile. I asked him what his name was and he looked away. Finally I asked him who I was, because it just hurt too much to think he wouldn't know. He looked straight into my eyes and said, "My Wife!" in a really hoarse voice and with a smile. I laughed out loud. I knew he would be okay and I knew I would be okay. He was still in there. Somewhere. He would come back eventually.

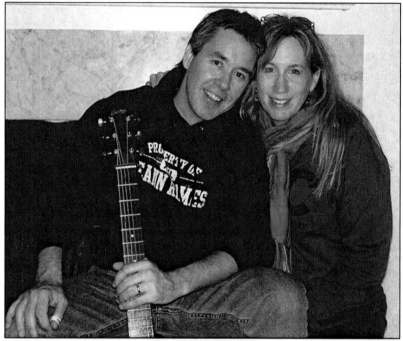

Pete and Erin in 2006

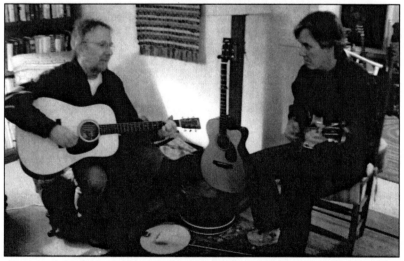

Pete and performer Herb Pedersen. Herb came by the house to help
Pete work on his guitar skills following the stroke.

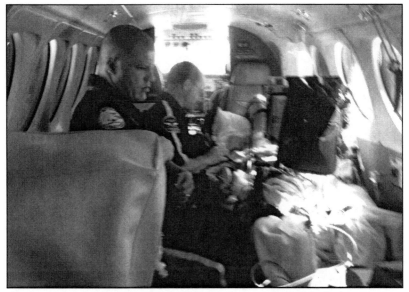

Pete on Vanderbilt University Medical Center's LifeFlight being sent to Texas Heart Institute, in Houston, Texas.

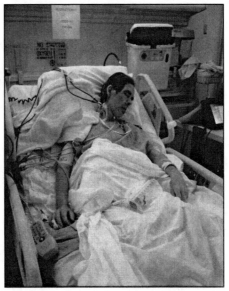

Two weeks following surgery.

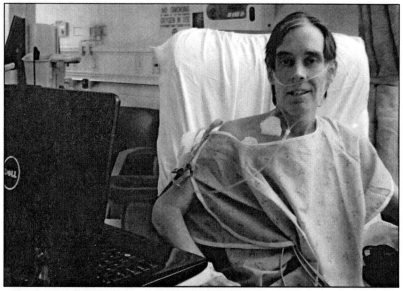

Trying to smile.

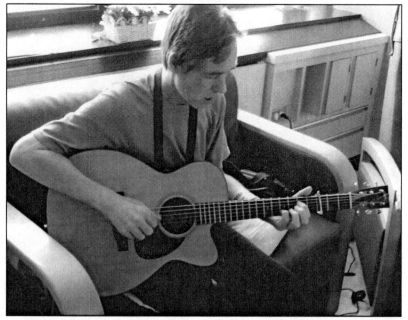

Pete's first attempt to play guitar after the heart surgery.

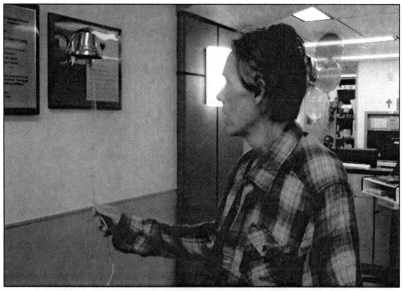

Ringing the bell as we were discharged from Texas Heart Institute.

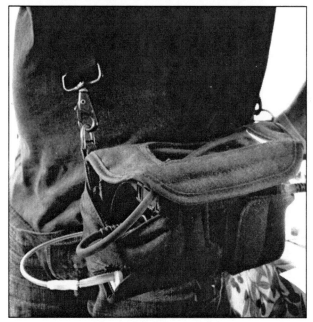

HeartWare™ device

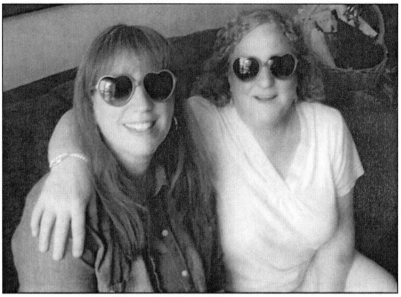

Erin and cousin Cath in Houston. Cath brought the heart-shaped glasses to add some levity to our day.

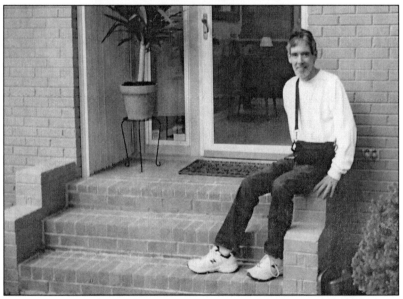

Our first day back at home in Nashville.

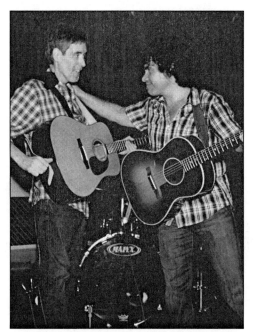

Pete performs "Leaving On A Jet Plane" with John Oates at the benefit.

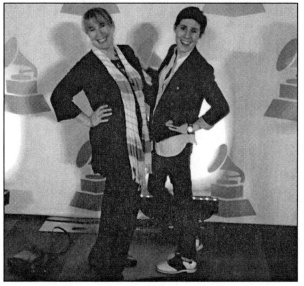

Erin and Sean striking a silly pose at a Grammy party.

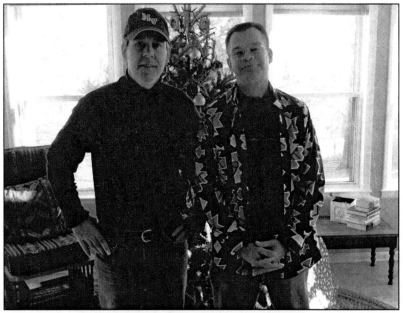

Pete and Carl – Christmas 2010 in Nashville

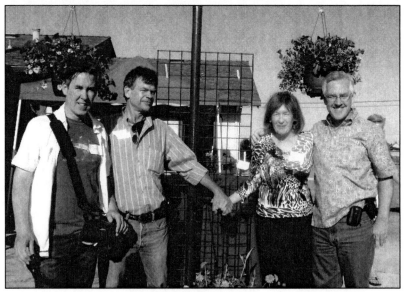

Pete, Carl, T and Frank

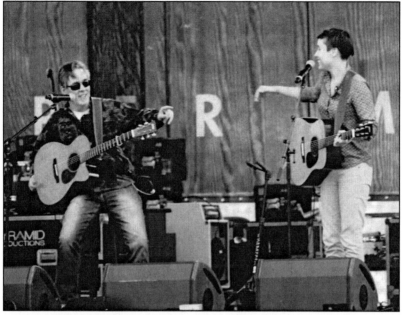

Pete and Sean on stage at Copper Mountain - 2013

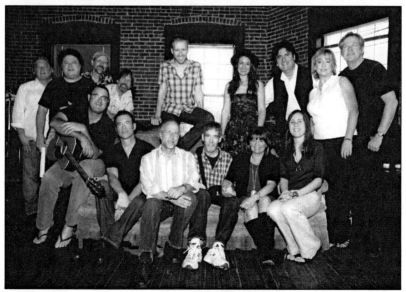

The cast of the benefit

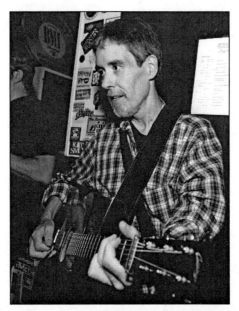

Pete getting ready to go on stage

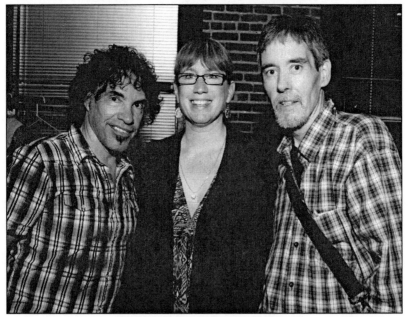

John Oates, Erin and Pete

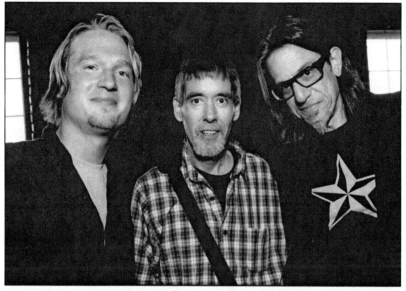

Jason Henke, Pete and Scott Goldman

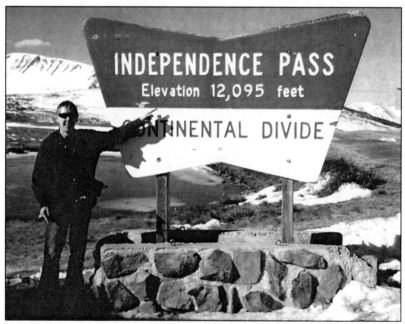

Pete at Independence Pass, CO 2012

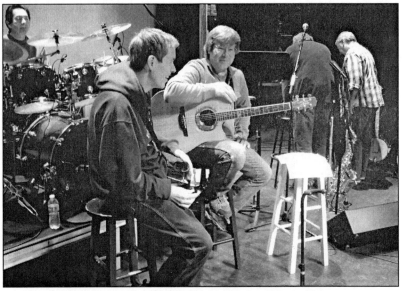

Pete sits in on stage at The Wheeler Opera House
for The John Denver Tribute show. L-R Richie Gajate-Garcia,
Pete, Jim Curry, Jim Horn, Herb Pedersen

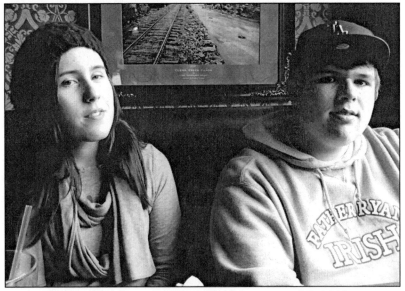

Sean and James at Hotel Jerome in Aspen, CO 2009

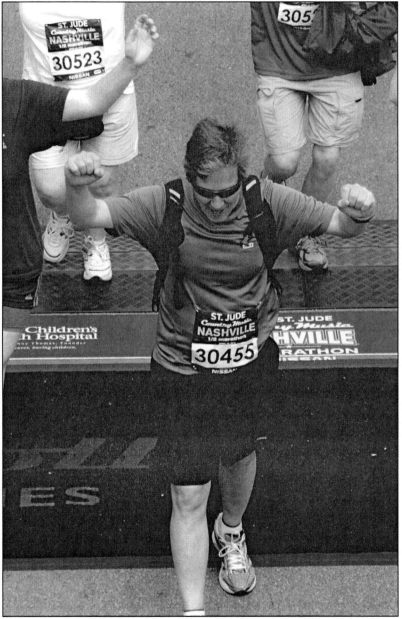

Crossing the finish line of the half-marathon
one year after being life-flighted to Houston, TX.

Pete Huttlinger and Erin Morris Huttlinger

Chapter Nine

A Journey Through ICU Psychosis

(So *That's* Where He Was)

Erin

Pete's psychosis while in ICU was lengthy and traumatizing. After he came out of it he told me about events that he was sure had happened. I tried but could not convince him that he had dreamt it all. The

111

fact that I "acted" like I didn't know what he was talking about added to his overall paranoia. At first I kind of laughed at him and thought it was funny until I realized how serious he was. It is something that he has had to really work through. Over the next few months following the surgery he slowly revealed his "dreams" to me. And to this day I still think there's a part of him that really believes these events ("journeys") happened. They were as much a part of his time in Houston as the real-life day-to-day events were to me.

Pete

I say "journeys" because there were many. I went to many places. I hosted a TV show. I visited with many people I knew, worked covert missions with some that I did not and protected friends of mine who wanted to get involved in them. I drove cattle to the hospital in Texas in the middle of the night. I helped protect a rare bee in a South American country for an old friend who had married a billionaire yet she still lived in a quiet little home in Nashville. I rescued my mom and my aunt Patty who had both been kidnapped.

When you are just lying in bed all day and all night on pain medicine and medicine for your heart, medicine for your lungs, medicine for your liver and medicine for your kidneys, you've got a lot of spare time on your hands (or, in my case, my back). The mind is such a powerful force within us it can take us away from pain and put us in a joyful spot or a dangerous place or a place full of wonder. It can literally deliver us smack dab in the middle of something so farfetched that you must be dreaming and then convince yourself beyond any shadow of a doubt that you were not. It is a great occupier of time.

Then, in what seemed like months but in fact, was only a couple of weeks later, I began to realize that it was just possible that I had been dreaming because my aunt Patty had passed away many years before I got sick. And then a couple of days later I remembered that my mom too, had passed away over ten years ago! I felt sad for her loss and that I did not even remember that she had died. What kind of a son forgets that his mother has passed away? A very sick kind of son.

My God! Was it all a dream? Had all these things not happened to me?

I do know that it was several months before I disclosed it all to Erin. We were lying in our bed in the hotel about a week before my final discharge from THI. It was about midnight and I finally felt comfortable enough to tell her where I had been during those days. It was very rare for me to be up so late at night. I was sleeping a lot back then. I would wake up in the morning, try to eat a little bit of cereal and then go back to bed and sleep for a couple of hours. Then I would rise again, try a little lunch and back to bed. Erin would try her best to get me up, have me sit in a chair, watch a little TV or try to read a book. (That brought on its own problems because I was on so many meds that my vision was messed up. I just couldn't focus on anything.) Then I would have something very small for dinner and then back to bed for the night. I would wait for the sun to set then I'd make a beeline for the bed. So being up at midnight was a rare thing for me.

I remember asking her, "Okay sweetie, do you want to know where I was?" She knew exactly what I was talking about. She's uncanny in that sense. And she replied, "Yes, if you're ready to tell me."

TV with LeAnn

The first place I went was so real to me that I was sure Erin was just not paying attention. She was there with me and she didn't even remember anything about it. "What a knucklehead," I thought. This is what ICU Psychosis can do. It can take you to a new place or an old place. Familiar surroundings or new and strange ones. This one was familiar to me and with friendly people that I thought a lot of.

Ten days after my surgery I co-hosted a TV show with LeAnn Rimes. Except for the fact that I just had major surgery, this was not out of the realm of possibility since I had worked with her on a number of shows and although she was not aware of what a great co-host I could be, I knew I could do it. And also LeAnn had phoned me at my house a few weeks before I went in to the hospital and asked me if I could do a gig with her. I suspected it was for her wedding because she wouldn't tell me much about the gig and the word was out that she was getting married. I had to turn her down because I was supposed to be a band leader on a gig at the Colorado Music Hall Of Fame that would be inducting John Denver into its hall. So it made sense that she had found out and asked me to do the TV show with her and there I was. (In reality, I never heard from LeAnn again after I turned down her gig.)

The TV show was taped at the Opryland Hotel in Nashville, Tennessee. We opened with a great number with the band playing and LeAnn came in dancing over some rocks that stuck up through a very small waterfall and into a very shallow river. It was very classy, looked great on TV and the audience at the taping loved it.

Next we went on to our first guest, Vince Gill. Vince is the guy everyone calls in Nashville whenever they need someone who is a great singer, great guitarist, funny interview subject and just an all-around great guy. Well, sure enough Vince noticed that I was in the same clothes I was wearing when I entered the hospital ten days prior. (I hadn't had time to get a change of clothes since I was coming right from the hospital to the TV taping. Heart surgery can really complicate things.) So we were supposed to play the next song with Vince but he covered for me and did the song without me while I ran off the set to get some clothes.

My next appearance on the show I was to interview guests Chris Hillman and Herb Pedersen. They had just flown in to Nashville and came directly from the airport to the taping. It turned out that Chris was feeling too tired and so Herb said, "No problem Pal, I'll take care of it for you." But I found myself a little bit taken aback by Herb's full head of bleached blonde hair and his new teeth. A whole new set of pearly white choppers. That was all I could see when I looked at him during our interview. His teeth were so white just like all the folks on TV these days that get the overlays or ultra-whitening done. I had to hold back a chuckle. It was very disconcerting since I had known Herb for thirteen or fourteen years at the time and I'd have thought he would have let me know if he were to make such a radical change.

(It was nice to see Herb in "real life" a few months after I got out of the hospital and saw that his naturally declining hair line and his own teeth were intact.)

My good friend Steve Emley was there at the TV taping. He's the first guy I met in Nashville that I could truly be myself with. I remember one night I was up till 3 a.m. writing a string arrangement for a jingle I was recording the next day. Then at 6 a.m. I heard banging going on just over my head. My landlord had not told me that he was having a new roof put on the house. So I got in my car and drove to Steve's house. At the time I barely knew Steve but he seemed like a good guy and I needed sleep. His door was unlocked so I let myself in and went straight to his couch. I woke up a couple of hours later when he walked in the room and said, "What are you doing here?" with a bit of wonderment in his voice. I told him what happened and we've been friends ever since.

He was not working on the TV show but he's the kind of guy who has a knack for showing up just when I need him. I was looking for some food and found out that I had missed my meal with the crew but that the hotel would gladly give me something for $20.00. I was livid. I was hosting a TV show in their hotel and the thought of them charging me for a meal really set me off. This probably dates back to the days when I used to play guitar in the hotel and we'd have to pay a king's ransom to park our cars so I was probably holding a little bit of a grudge. Steve found me some food. All was well.

After the show I saw LeAnn and told her that I thought everything went pretty well. She agreed and we said goodbye. There was no mention of my wardrobe mistake. I figured it must have happened to her from time to time.

Well, then it was time to go home. I had no ride but a crewmember said he'd take me home if I didn't mind waiting. My chest was a little sore but I said I'd wait just the same. He came to get me and he had a plate of food covered to take home. For some reason it was a Thanksgiving meal. This was in May. The mind is a powerful thing. He got on the highway but he was going the wrong direction. I don't mean that he was headed north in the southbound lane. He was going east and I wanted to go west. Back to Texas.

The next thing I remember was waking up in my hospital bed in Houston and telling Erin about the TV show. She said something like, "No honey. That never happened. I think I'd remember that." I wrote her off as a complete nut case. Obviously I had just hosted a TV show with LeAnn Rimes. Didn't she see it on TV? I was just there. It was great. I played with LeAnn on the opener and closer. Left the stage for Vince's spot and returned to interview our friend

Herb. I kept trying to convince her that I had hosted the show with LeAnn but she must not have been feeling well because she couldn't remember it ever happening. It did not matter to me that I was the one in bed strapped down, with IV's coming out of my arms, and a catheter to help me urinate, and various tubes going in and out of my body to help move some blood around. I had just been to Nashville and co-hosted a TV show with LeAnn Rimes.

The Military

My next journey was a very interesting one in which I would exit the hospital and board a plane at midnight at an old abandoned airport in Houston. This one continues to haunt me because too many things surrounding it kept reinforcing the fact that it could have happened.

It was a military plane. Fully equipped with lots of guns and ammunition, lots of medicine and medics on hand and sleeper bunks.

Now I am not a gun person. I don't like them or what they do to people every single day in America. But for some reason I had been contacted and asked if I would do something for my country and I said, "Yes."

I would board the plane along with two or three other "recruits" like me. We would get our military gear on: boots, pants, flak jackets with bulletproof vests, gloves, and helmets. The whole time we were getting geared up, we were being briefed on our mission and the plane would be taking off down the runway to our destination: a South American country and one time a Middle Eastern country.

This took place very shortly after my surgery. I know this because in the ICU where I was being treated there were glass doors separating the patients and it allowed the nurses to keep an eye on more of us. This was really unnecessary because I had one and only one nurse at a time at my bedside day and night. Twenty-four hours a day.

One night we had injured a man we were after. This man was a big and very dark skinned African-American. He had been hit in the hand and he had lost a finger. I believe it was his right hand pinky finger.

Well, the man in the room that I could see from my bed was a very large African-American man. His hand appeared to be band-aged. I was more than certain that this was not a dream. It was real.

We couldn't speak to anyone about the operations we were going on either during or after we had completed our missions. Those were part of the rules or conditions we had agreed to.

So now I'm lying in a bed in a hospital not thirty feet from a man who had been injured in our recent operation. I was certain he was going to kill me. But now the problem was that I couldn't speak because there was a tube down my throat and I couldn't move because I was either strapped to the bed or the drugs were so strong I couldn't move. I could not tell which. To say that I was feeling a little stressed would be putting it more than a little lightly.

We would each lie in our beds, our eyes set on each other. I would stare at him and wonder when he was going to get out of his bed and come into my room and kill me. Then night would come again and off I'd go. Back to the abandoned airfield and on to the airplane.

The Middle East

On one mission I was deployed to the Middle East. I don't know what country I was in and I don't think I was ever told but

I was there to infiltrate the locals and stop them from harming the "good guys." I had two old friends who were interested in joining me in my midnight missions. Lee from Virginia and Steve from Nashville. We had many adventures together in our younger days in Nashville and Lee had been into some kind of reality show at the time that took people out on the very type of missions I was on. But the difference was that mine were "real" missions with "real" bullets and "real" blood. I didn't want my friends to get hurt so I convinced Steve to tell Lee that I just couldn't make it happen. He understood what I was saying: I could make it happen but it would be best for them if they weren't involved.

I had met a family and fallen for the daughter of the house. She was very pretty and very naïve. She had two or three brothers. It was always hard to tell because the brothers always had friends over and I had a hard time telling who was part of the family and who was not. It was not good for me to ask too many questions.

We were in a very small village in the middle of nowhere. There was a very long and very straight road coming into and out of the village. To the west there was a hill and there were cheaply made bunkers where snipers would hide. They would seemingly shoot at anyone who was not them. How they could tell the difference from such a vantage point I never knew. On the good side of things was the fact that this village was so remote that almost no one ever came by there.

To the east it was desert as far as you could see. The flat terrain never varied. The sun was hot. People mostly stayed in during the days. The male children went to school. Though the girl I was interested in was home schooled. Her family was progressive but very cautious. They did not approve of me but somehow I managed to convince them I was one of them. I look nothing like a Middle Eastern man so this is still an area of concern for me.

How in the world did I convince them that I, a fair-skinned man, was good enough for their lovely daughter?

At night the little village came to life. Stores opened up. People were out in the streets. It was pleasant but there was a cloud of uneasiness over everyone. I couldn't put my finger on it but there seemed to be a local power struggle going on. I spoke the language fluently so there were no communication issues surrounding me. The family that I was associated with and subsequently stayed with had an actual maze that entrants had to get through in order to get into their house.

You would first enter a ten-foot gated wall that was padlocked. Then you would be directed to a maze of turns — right, left then right again before you would arrive at the front door. All the while walls that were eight to ten feet high surrounded you. Your sense of direction was always being thrown off. That was the kind of protection every house in this little village had. No one was to come in who was not welcomed.

One night I was out and a rival gang of the family where I was staying caught me. We were at a little market store and I went in to purchase something. The man behind the counter made me almost immediately and discovered that I had a gun, which was illegal in this town. Virtually every male over ten years old had one so why it was illegal? I never knew. But it was and I was caught. Perhaps it was only illegal for people who were not from the village to have one. I was made to get in their car with a bunch of young and heavily armed men with scarves covering their faces, but somehow I managed to escape and get to my family's house where I was promptly disowned by the family as soon as they heard I was in trouble. I discovered that the girl's older brother was the one who had outed me at the store. He never liked me but I didn't know just how much until then. The look on his face was one of hatred. The kind of look only the youth get when they are caught between right and wrong. Knowing that they are wrong but they are too young to admit it. Caught in a precipice between wanting to love someone, even as a friend, and staying true to your family history, the ways of your people and survival. That look is stuck in my memory.

The girl, his sister, refused to speak to me.

I had to escape town immediately and get to my contact, who was hiding near the bunkers on the hill to the west, and then next thing I knew I was back on the plane headed to Houston. Back to the Texas Heart Institute.

Osama bin Laden was killed in Abbottabad, Pakistan on May 2nd 2011, two days before my surgery. I was in a state of constant pain and on a wonderful morphine drip. This may have had something to do with the previous story.

Frank and Pete's excellent adventure(s)

My brother Frank is a fantastic guy. Always ready to go to a museum or to a clock store or to an antique store. And that is great if you are into museums, clocks or antiques. Now don't get me wrong, I like them all but not quite as much as Frank does. That never stops him.

"Pete, do you need another clock?" Frank says.

"No thanks." I reply.

"Would you like to go to a museum?" He says.

"How about lunch instead?" I say. "I'll buy."

"Sounds good to me. Then we'll go to a museum." He says.

He's always been fun to be around and he's always been the kind of brother who looked after his younger brother. When we were kids in Virginia I recall going out to play with him and some other kids in the neighborhood. Because of my heart condition I could never keep up. "Wait for me," I would call out. He'd turn and say, "C'mon Pete. You can do it." I couldn't but I would always try and I appreciated his encouragement.

One day when we were in high school (I was a freshman and Frank a junior), a group of guys threw something at me as I was walking past them. I think it was an apple but it could have just as easily been a rock. I was shy and a bit of a loner so I didn't really know how to handle it. That night I mentioned to Frank what had happened. He asked me what I had done to make them want to throw something at me. I told him I had done nothing. When he was convinced, he said simply, "I'll take care of it."

The next evening at home Frank said to me, "Those guys won't be bothering you again." I never asked and he never offered. I walked by them a few days later just to make sure. They left me alone. No more rocks. No more apples.

So it was no surprise when Frank and his wife, Wendy, were already at the hospital in Houston waiting for me when I arrived. He was obviously concerned and I, being the younger brother, tried to make light of the situation. When I was able to speak I would joke about all the Viagra that I was taking. Three times a day makes even a very sick man hard as a rock. At least if I was going to die, it would be with a smile on my face.

On the day of my surgery Frank, T and Erin stood around me and held hands while Frank offered up a prayer. It was a beautiful prayer that later spoke volumes to me about Frank and who he'd become in the years since we were kids. He liked to drink beer, ride motorcycles, and go to museums, concerts and clock stores. He loved his kids and his entire extended family and in that moment I knew he loved me too.

So the following events, which took place in the middle of the night outside of Houston, came as no surprise to me.

Frank and I would take a tractor-trailer rig far out of town to a remote area and when we arrived at our destination, the trailer would be loaded with cattle by a group of men who appeared to be Mexican but they could just as well have been Americans. Calves and younger cattle. No older ones were taken. The trailer was split into two levels. The lower one was where the younger calves were and the upper was for the older and bigger cows. The truck would be loaded by one in the morning then things got a little tricky.

For some reason we could not both ride in the cab of the truck so Frank would have to ride in the trailer with the cows. He'd get undressed, and then he would take a drug that would slow his breathing to protect him from the methane fumes that all the cattle put out. The drug also put him to sleep. Then I would drive for a couple of hours and when I stopped for refueling I would wake Frank, get him some oxygen and food, give him more drugs and out to sleep he'd go.

Then we'd arrive back at the Texas Heart Institute. I pulled into a circular drive entrance at the lowest level of the hospital. We would drive around and around in several circles going up slowly one floor at a time. Once there, people showed up and jumped into action. The first thing they did was get Frank out of the truck, revive him and get him some food again.

They would give him a much-needed shower to clean off all of the manure that the cattle had showered him with during the drive. Then they carefully unloaded all of the cattle where they did medical experiments on them. Then they would finally attend to me, get me back to the hospital bed and hook me back up to all the machines and get out again before the nurses noticed anything.

The next night we were out again. I wasn't feeling very good because I'd just had surgery, so instead of switching roles Frank agreed that he'd go in with the cattle again. This time, however, our uncle Frank Walker joined me for the ride. (Why could I take a passenger with me on the second night but not the first? Hey, that's the power of drugs.) Uncle Frank was in his mid-80's so he wouldn't be driving, but he was great with a map and we appeared to be headed to a different locale on this night. I was happy to have him with me.

We got to the ranch, loaded the cattle, drugged Frank and put him in the trailer. Off we went. I was driving which was not that unbelievable since when I was eighteen I worked for the U.S. Forest Service at Croatan National Forest in eastern North Carolina. While there, the older guys taught me to drive a tractor-trailer. It was actually fun.

When we stopped for gas there was some kind of commotion and in the melee we forgot to get to Frank, wake him, feed him, drug him and put him back with the cattle. So by the time I remembered about Frank we were almost back at THI and I was yelling for him to hang on. "Hang in there, Franco!" I hollered, not knowing if he could hear me or not. "We're almost there!" Uncle Frank didn't seem worried and that helped.

When we finally arrived, we rushed to get Frank out, wake him and get some fluid into him. I apologized for not getting to him. Explained what had happened. He looked me in the eye and said matter-of-factly, "Peter, I have done this twice for you. I'm not doing it again." He said it with such finality in his tone that I knew our adventures for THI were over.

The Bees

Carolyn was a neighbor of mine in Nashville many years ago. She had since divorced her husband, Michael, and re-married a billionaire whose name I never got. Although she was married to a man who had untold wealth she never let it be known that she had money. She moved to a different house in our quiet neighborhood. It had a beautiful sunroom and lots and lots of flowers inside and outside of the house. She had developed a love of bees. Strange I know. But not to Carolyn. She enjoyed watching them pollinate the flowers. She was completely unafraid of them and, most importantly, she was on a mission.

She approached me one evening. Not in the hospital. It was somewhere else. I don't know where. But she found me just the same. She asked me if I would take a trip with her to South America to rescue some bees. I can recall thinking that she must have been off her rocker because bees don't need rescuing. They can simply fly away. She pointed out the rarity of a particular species of bee in South America and convinced me that I was the one she needed to help. She also told me that she could be a big help to my career with her husband's contacts. So I agreed to help.

It was just one trip to South America but what a trip it was. Carolyn and I got on her private jet and flew all night. We arrived in mid-morning the next day, had a bite to eat, laid low and slept until dusk. We got up and suddenly we were transformed to a place of such supernatural beauty that I had a hard time concentrating on the task at hand. I remember a river and flowers at the edge of it. It was like something from a Disney movie. We worked our way to a place that jutted out over the water. We had to reach very far to get one of the bees. One was all we needed. We got him.

Then suddenly we were in a city and the next thing I knew Carolyn was on top of a woman with a gun in her hand. The woman was dealing drugs and Carolyn did not approve. She threatened the woman. The woman threatened her. Carolyn told her who her husband was and the woman quieted down quickly. Carolyn beat the woman and then we were back on the plane. While on the trip back to Nashville, Carolyn told me what was really going on.

She was suffering, dying actually, from a rare disease. There was no cure and she had come to terms with it. She would get tired occasionally and would get the rest she needed. Her billionaire husband understood that she was on a mission to save the bees and to be left alone to die. That was why she lived alone in Nashville and he lived elsewhere.

The next thing I knew we were at a large awards show. I was to perform there but I was not nominated for anything! I didn't know what or why I was supposed to perform. As it turned out Carolyn was the guest of honor at this wonderful function. She had arranged for me to perform there because there were so many movers and shakers in the music biz that would be in atten-

dance. I was prepared with a great guitar instrumental number but it didn't matter because by the time I performed, no one was paying any attention. It was more of an embarrassment to me than anything. She swore that she would make it up to me. I told her that I was okay and thanked her for trying to help my career and I told her that maybe I should have a reason to be there the next time.

Then she needed to go home suddenly to get some rest. I never saw Carolyn again.

I woke up at THI again.

My mom and Aunt Patty

They were just two kind, older ladies in their 70's who wanted to try and save a few helpless dogs. Nothing either of them had ever experienced a desire to do in the past.

They grew up as sisters in a Catholic family of six children in San Francisco. Three boys and three girls. Then they got older. My mom married and had seven boys and one girl. Aunt Patty had four boys and seven girls. All of Aunt Patty's girl's first names were Mary. There was very little time for dogs. So that they would be involved in such an adventure was nothing short of amazing, even though Aunt Patty did get into stand-up comedy at age 70!

I don't know how it started but they had been involved in some kind of animal rescue. They were in the northwestern part of the United States. But suddenly they weren't. They were in Mexico and we were deployed to break them free from their captors. But this was my own mother and my aunt! How could I be involved? How could I not? Then, just as fast, we were back in the northeast.

Crawling through something. I don't know what. Things were moving too fast. I couldn't keep up. Mom needed me. Aunt Pat needed me. It was all so confusing.

Then I awakened to find that my cousins George and Joe were coming to visit me in the hospital. It was late May or early June. I was touched that they would come to visit me and I was told that they were on their way home from Florida and they wanted to stop by. I asked why they were in Florida and was told they were on a road trip. George and Joe on a road trip to Florida and the way home was through Houston, Texas? Now I was more than convinced that all the places I'd been, all the adventures I'd had were not dreams at all. They had to be true.

George was a captain in the Navy. He was a decorated California law enforcement officer. He also worked for the Department of Justice. He was very well connected. Joe, his younger brother, had traveled to Africa a couple of years prior to meet George for a "vacation." "Yeah right." Like I'm going to believe that after all the places I've been the past month. The cattle in the middle of the night. The LeAnn Rimes TV show. The covert missions. The Middle East. The bee rescue. And now my mom and Aunt Patty? Their own mother? These guys were involved and deeply so. I had to let them know that everything was okay. I had to remind them that my mom and their mom had passed away ten and twelve years before respectively. I had to let them know.

The only problem was that I had not yet been out of bed. Since my arrival in Houston over one month ago. I had not been out of bed. I couldn't move. There were all these damned IV's and tubes coming out of my body. I was strapped down at times. I had a feeding tube down my nose for God's sake! I couldn't have done any of these things or been to any of these places. But I had. The memories were and still are as real as the keyboard I'm writing this on. I had done these things and been to these places. As of this writing it has been almost three years and the memories are just as vivid today as they were then.

George and Joe arrived just after the hospital staff got me out of bed for the first time in over a month. They sat me in a chair and I was excited to see them. I was down to 110 lbs. from my normal 165 lbs. I'm sure I looked like an Auschwitz victim though I hadn't seen myself yet. I hadn't showered in five weeks. All the bathing I'd had had been done while still laying down by nurses and staff at Texas Heart Institute.

So there I sat in the chair when George and Joe arrived. The ghost inside of me looked out at them and tried to smile. I didn't rise to greet them because I couldn't. It would still be weeks before I could stand on my own. They must have been horrified when they saw me but their laughter is always their strongest point and they managed to laugh out loud. I tried to question them quietly, without actually calling it what it was, about the mission they were on but they only gave me vague answers. I was more convinced with each response. A road trip from Florida to California? That didn't make any sense. What were they trying to tell me? I couldn't make sense of it.

So I told them I was tired, put my head down on the tray table where I was seated and went to sleep. I couldn't keep my head up any longer and I obviously wasn't able to get through to my cousins.

My last journey was a very strange one indeed. I was at someone's house in Northern California or Northern Italy. Nothing was clear in my mind any longer. They both make great wines.

What else could the connection be? I had lived in Northern California as a kid but I had traveled to Northern Italy just the year before. I remember a map of the area and while I never saw them, there were guards that protected us.

Us?
Who was with me?
I don't know.
There was a lot of brush around the house. Low brush. And a long road that wound through the hills to get to the house. It was not an easy place to find.

It was a comfortable house with lots of windows on one side that opened up to a patio of sorts that had beautiful flowers growing all around it. But just as soon as you got to the property line, which was quite some distance, the flowers were no longer in view.

The inside had a fair amount of clutter. Paintings were done by the owner and they hung on the walls. I was staying at someone's house and it was time for me to go.

All my belongings were packed and ready and though I didn't want to, I had to leave. It was time for me to go to the next part of my journey. I didn't know where I was going. But the boxes were packed and labeled and I was out the door. The map I had made no sense. I couldn't find my way out of the winding hills. The roads I took made no sense to me. But I kept trying until finally I woke up – again.

Back in the hospital room at THI.

Chapter Ten

The Recovery

Erin

I can't live without the love of people around me. But I'm a solitary person. I need a lot of time by myself especially if I'm in problem solving mode. I had so many offers from family and close friends to come to Houston to sit with me over the months. The offers came from people I love and need. But except in cases where they were spotting me so I could go home to Nashville for a few days and see the kids, I, politely I hope, declined their offers.

One of my coping mechanisms, I've noticed, is to create rituals in every new situation. Then I pattern my day around those rituals. They keep me very calm and very focused. And when days are long and stressful, it gives me something to look forward to. It's something I can control and gives me small rewards throughout the day. I'm not at all obsessive/compulsive about these rituals but as I've pondered it, I realize that if there are other people around me, it makes it very difficult to observe those rituals. I tend to be focused on other people's needs and often lock myself into whatever their stresses might be. I absorb other people's anxieties and worries and mine get shoved out of the way. And during this time, the only people whose stresses I was most concerned about were Pete, Sean and James. I didn't have room for much more.

So having even the most wonderfully supportive people around can sometimes short circuit me. I see this as my own flaw, not theirs. Nobody in our families was demanding anything of me, or asked me for anything. I just have a very, very focused energy especially during traumatic times. And for me, that requires concentrated focus and a certain amount of solitude.

Here's an outline of my rituals on an average day in Houston while Pete was hospitalized. Visiting hours began at 8 a.m. So I was up, showered and out of the hotel by 7:45 most mornings. I would walk the two blocks to the hospital. Most of the time it was brutally hot, but I would try to enjoy the fact that I could get out and see the blue sky and summer flowers. And there was a bridge I would cross on the way. I would stop and watch the fish swimming in the shallow stream. Pete and I love to fly fish so I would imagine that we would be doing that again someday. Once

I got to the hospital I would head straight to McDonalds (which is a completely upsetting thing to see in a place where people are being cured of a lot of the illnesses that fast food triggers.) I would get a grotesquely large Diet Coke to fuel me for hours. (I have since broken myself of this habit. I'm sure it was killing me slowly and I don't want to ever be sick.) I would head up to Pete's room in ICU with my backpack loaded down with my laptop, iPad, phone, all my chargers and files full of work. Then I'd set up shop in the hospital for the day. I would take 15 minute breaks throughout the day and hit the cafeteria. I was such a regular there for so many months that sometimes the cashiers would give me the employee discount since they were sure I must actually work somewhere in the hospital.

The hospital would kick everyone out during shift change between 6:00-8:00 p.m. So I would head out the back door of the hospital, across the street into an office building and head up to the 6th floor to Trevisio — a wonderful restaurant with a great happy hour and the sweetest hostess and bartenders. I would order a happy hour glass of wine, some light dinner and read a book – usually Benjamin Franklin, a biography written by Walter Isaacson. I'd read it several times before, so I could just open it anywhere and read something interesting and leave it at that. I was not able to get engrossed in any books because my mind just couldn't stay focused long enough. At 8pm, I'd head back to the hospital and sit with Pete until 10pm when they'd make me leave. So two blocks back to the hotel, over the bridge with one eye over my shoulder all the time watching for any danger signs, then up to my efficiency hotel room. At that point I'd have another glass of wine, try to relax, write on CaringBridge (an online journal that allows caregivers to post health updates) and watch television. I was often awake until 1 or 2 in the morning just trying to de-stress from the day.

So that was the cocoon I'd built around myself. I got so locked into this way of life while we were in Houston that re-entry back into everyday life in Nashville took some adjustment. I could no longer indulge myself in this over-simplified, secluded lifestyle.

There was a huge sigh of relief among family and doctors that Pete had successfully survived the surgery. But I was quickly becoming aware that one accomplishment achieved brought another hurdle to jump. Each day went by much like the day before. Progress seemed slower than slow, but I realize now that Pete wasn't just recovering from open-heart surgery. He was recovering from months of a slow, near-death event and open-heart surgery. It was not going to be a quick healing process.

I was concerned about Pete not being communicative and that the ICU psychosis seemed to be lingering too long. All I could think about was what if he'd had another stroke during the surgery. I guess I finally worried the doctors enough that they agreed to do a CT scan of his brain. Fortunately it came back as all clear. The real hurdle though was waiting for Pete's kidney's to "wake up" as the doctors called it. The kidneys were traumatized and had shut down before Pete's surgery, along with his liver and stomach. But the kidneys seemed to have everyone concerned. He was checked several times a day by the kidney team of doctors. At first they said not to worry, that it could take up to four or five days. He was put on dialysis regularly and after a few days I could see that the doctors were looking a little bit puzzled. So we waited. In the meantime, the nurses worked tirelessly to make Pete comfortable and to build his strength.

By then it had been nearly five weeks since Pete had eaten any solid food. I'm not sure what the theory was on the doctor's end of things, but nobody seemed overly concerned about it. Eventually after enough pleading from me, they inserted a feeding tube. This may have been part of their plan all along, but I just couldn't get a handle on it and the doctors weren't in a hurry or at least not in enough of a hurry for me.

After the feeding tube was threaded through his nose and down into his stomach, they started giving him liquid food ever so slowly. And I could see why. The slightest bit too much and it would come right back up. All his organs still weren't functioning as they should and they could only tolerate so much.

One day, I went to get some lunch. I was gone about 30 minutes and when I returned I noticed that the feeding tube had been moved to Pete's other nostril. When I questioned the nurse, she said that Pete had pulled it out and they had to reinsert it. He had no idea what he was doing; he just knew he wanted it out. The next day the same thing happened and then he started pulling on his IVs in his arm. I felt so bad for him because I didn't know what was going on in his mind, but at that point he had to be restrained. The nurses strapped his arms to the side of his bed to keep him from hurting himself. If I was sitting with him and keeping an eye on things, they'd take them off. This only lasted about 48 hours until he stopped trying to set himself free from all the tubes.

Meanwhile, his kidneys just sat there. Nothing. So we waited.

I couldn't bear the thought of leaving Pete, but I was starting to get very stressed about the kids. I couldn't wait any longer. I needed to get home to see them and to let them see me. It was summer and there was nothing going on for them school-wise.

They were fending for themselves and spending time with my family. And every time my family offered to come to Houston and be with me, I just told them that what I needed most was for them to occupy Sean and James and help them keep the house together.

So I took advantage of the fact that Pete was in his own dream world and bought a round trip ticket for Nashville. Cath Strong, Pete's cousin, Frank and Wendy, all flew back to Houston to cover for me for a few days.

I barely remember what happened over those few days at home, just that I was elated to see the kids and I'm sure the feeling was mutual. The whole family tried to get quiet time together and I did some bookkeeping things that needed to be done. But the time just went too quickly and we were so sad to separate again.

While I was gone, Pete came out of his fog. I was delivered a message via an email from Pete. Cath had opened up an iPad for Pete and he was able to type a cryptic message, "Hi Sweetie." I was so happy to know that Pete would be able to talk to me once I got back to Houston. Another hurdle jumped.

When I returned to Houston, the family had gone back to their respective homes. Pete seemed happy to see me.

Slowly Pete was helped to sit up in bed, then eventually he was helped to a reclining chair. I'll never forget seeing his back for the first time in a month. He was skin and bones. Down to 110 pounds from his normal 165. He already looked like an 80-year-old man in the face, but when I saw his back through the split in the gown as they sat him up on the side of the bed, I was dumbstruck. He looked like a holocaust survivor. A ribcage with a layer of thin skin covering it. I was careful not to let Pete see the shock on my face. All I could think of was if he saw himself he would be so depressed. Fortunately there weren't mirrors and even if there were he wasn't particularly interested.

From the edge of the bed, to the chair. And within a couple of days, from the chair to a walker. It was time for Pete to try and walk. I'm not exaggerating when I say that it took five minutes for the two physical therapists just to get Pete safely from the bed to the chair. His equilibrium was off since he'd been flat for so many weeks. He was highly unstable and could barely even lift his foot to turn himself around. They had to give him instructions how to move his body. It was like he'd completely forgotten how to move.

The physical therapists put straps around him so they could keep a strong grip on him as he tried to take some steps with the walker. We left his ICU room and moved toward the nurse's station a few feet away. I followed closely with a wheelchair and after just a few steps, he would sit down. Then stand up and repeat. The encouragement the nurses and therapists gave him was fantastic. Applause rang out after only 25 steps down the hall. Of course, he was wheeled back to his room, too tired to make the return trip on his own power.

But his kidneys were still not working, even as his other vital signs were showing improvement. So we waited.

Soon, after he was able to walk about 100 steps, he was moved from ICU to 12 Tower. 12 Tower is a floor within the Texas Heart Institute that is dedicated to cardiac patients who are recovering from a transplant, or implantation of a special device. 12 Tower brought forth a slew of new nurses and procedures and again we adjusted. Pete began a more rigorous physical therapy routine. Daily he would be gotten out of bed, propped in front of his walker and led around the floor baby-stepping his way. Our conversations were still limited to what he needed, what he didn't need, what he didn't want and how he felt, how much he hated taking pills and how his food held zero interest. There were no smiles, none of his wonderful sense of humor. He was completely focused on himself. One of the doctors explained to me that he had no strength to offer me anything else. His body was so compromised that it took all of his energy just to live. There wasn't anything else. I began to wonder if I would ever hear him crack a joke again, or laugh loudly like he always had done. I decided to just be grateful that he was alive though it was getting harder and harder to remember the old Pete, the one I married who had such a lust for life and a wicked sense of humor.

Pete was starting to have to really work at things now. Up to this point, all the work was going on around him and he just had to keep breathing. Now the workload was shifting. He had to try and eat. He had to start swallowing pills instead of getting his medications intravenously. He had to try and sit up more and he had to try to walk. All this was beginning to stress him out and it showed on his face. He started to become more agitated. Eventually he called in some brotherly backup. Pete's brother Carl came for a visit.

Chapter Eleven

When The Going Gets Tough—The Tough Call Carl

Pete

When I was fourteen I found out that my father did not die of a heart attack as I had been led to believe. He killed himself. Suicide. I also found out at that time that my Grandmother on my mom's side killed herself on Christmas Day when mom was just sixteen years old. She took a gun and shot herself. Three weeks

139

after finding out those little tidbits, my brother Joe took his own life. Three weeks before I graduated from college, my brother Mike committed suicide. That's a lot of suicides for one family. Fifteen years after Mike died my cousin Alicia took her life but not before she killed her five year-old daughter, Jineva Belle.

So there you have it. The deepest, darkest secrets I have in my life. I've got nothing else to hide that would make any difference. And quite frankly, it feels good to put it in writing. The details surrounding each horrendous death are not important – interesting in a dark macabre kind of a way – but otherwise not helpful.

So that leaves me, Frank, Carl, and T. Carl and I were very close. At least I was as close as someone could be with Carl. When we moved from California to North Carolina in December of 1977, I was sixteen and Carl was twenty-one years old. We had fun driving out from California. It was a life-changing experience. A real adventure.

While we were in our new home, making new friends and learning our way around New Bern, N.C., I was trying to run a mile. I had never done this before in my life. I would get half way and then stop. Try again another day. One day in the spring of 1978 Carl decided to go with me. He was always encouraging me. That day I ran my first mile with Carl by my side. It was a special day in my life and I'm so grateful to Carl for his prodding me along, "You can do it, Pete."

Then six months after we moved to North Carolina, I was feeling homesick. Carl had some money so we borrowed mom's Volkswagen Bug and took off back to California for a little visit. I don't know if I had yet heard of Thomas Wolfe's book, "You Can't Go Home Again" but it was instantly clear to me that my old friends had gone on without me, my old town was getting along just fine without me and I felt like an outsider. Only six months had passed and I was a complete misfit.

So, after busting Carl out of jail, which he was in for some long-forgotten traffic violations, he and I headed back to North Carolina to continue our respective journeys. Usually together and usually full of mischief.

I was married to my first wife, Rhonda, when I was still in college. I couldn't find a way to pay for my last semester so I told mom and Carl that I would wrap things up and move to Nashville sooner than I had planned. Carl told me to get back to Boston and finish school. He paid for my last semester. Now, granted it didn't cost $25,000 for one semester back in 1984. I believe it was less than $2,000. Regardless, it was a lot of money for either of us.

When Carl got married he chose not to have a best man because I couldn't be there to fill the role.

So Carl and I were close. At one point we were tired of all the deaths in our family and so we made a pact. If either of us ever thought we would want to end our own lives, we would simply pick up the phone and call the other.

It was early to mid-June 2011. I was in Houston lying in the hospital bed, peeing on myself, crapping on myself unable to get out of bed, unable to eat anything at all without throwing up. Even the pills they would give me would be treated with such disrespect by my failing body that up they'd come within moments after taking them.

Carl had been admitted to a drug rehabilitation center in the desert outside of San Diego before I had been sent to Houston. He'd had a long battle with drug addiction. Well over twenty-five years' worth. It started when we were little kids. He would "huff" glue, he smoked a lot of pot and then after a bad motorcycle accident he got into pain killers and later on he turned to something called crank. He told me it was a poor man's version of crack. I made it clear to Carl and everyone else in my family that he was not to leave the rehab facility to come and visit me. (Picture the scene from the movie Young Frankenstein where the doctor goes in to see the monster and tells Inga and Igor not to open the door no matter what he does, no matter what he says.) It was important that he get the help he needed to get off drugs.

Erin had left for a week to go home to Nashville to be with Sean and James and my niece Molly came from New Orleans to be with me in the hospital. Erin never wanted me left completely alone.

Well, no sooner had Erin left and Molly arrived that I decided it was time to call in the big guns. I needed Carl. I didn't want to live like this any longer. I had neither the strength nor the means to do anything about it but I was scared at the thoughts I was having and I decided to make good on our pact. The phones were ringing off the hook from Houston; Nashville; Irvine, CA; Winona, MS; and San Diego. Erin called Frank. Frank called T. T called Molly. I called Carl.

I needed him to come and see me and I needed him now. The more everyone questioned me, the more determined I became. Everyone thought I had taken a long walk off a short pier and landed in the rabbit hole. ("Under any circumstances do not open this door" was ringing through Erin's head I'm sure. While my own version of "Don't you know a joke when you hear it?" was running through mine.)

Well, everyone made a deal with the rehab center. Three days was all he could have. Three days was all we would need. Carl arrived as Molly was leaving and we danced around the subject the first day. Carl acquainted himself with the hospital and met all the nurses, several doctors and lots of patients. Carl was great at meeting folks and it didn't matter who or where or what their situation was. He could meet anyone and within a few minutes leave an indelible mark on their lives.

The next day he said, "So, you called me here for a reason. What's up?" I told him that I was sick and tired of being sick and tired and I didn't want to continue this way. He listened and thought about it before saying that he understood and didn't blame me one bit for feeling this way. He also reminded me that things were going to get better; I'd just have to give it some time. And that was really all I needed. I just needed to tell Carl what I was feeling and he would talk me off the ledge.

Carl passed away February 7, 2014 from cancer. He phoned me two weeks before he died and said tearfully, "Hey Pete, remember when you called and you said 'I need you and I need you now?' Well, the tide has turned. I need you now, buddy." Erin and I went out to San Diego and we were able to visit with him right up until the end.

Chapter Twelve

A Birthday Gift

Erin

About this time Pete's kidneys "woke up." Just like that. All of a sudden. They weren't working, and then they were. Hallelujah! No more dialysis. The hope for a good recovery had just gotten better. All those involved heaved a huge sigh of relief. Slowly but surely all Pete's organs where cranking back up into action.

My new hurdle now was to focus on getting Pete to eat. He still couldn't eat without vomiting up half of it. He just wasn't in-

145

terested. I nudged him with his favorite foods, which as it turned out, he didn't have any favorites any more. He insisted that everything he put in his mouth just tasted like "dirt." I brought him ice cream, pie, candy bars, soda. Absolutely nothing appealed to him. We needed to help him build up his strength and good food was a part of this. But it was an uphill battle and Pete was in charge of this one. He would eat a few Cheerios here and there, maybe drink a carton of milk. His appetite was something that would build very slowly over time. But it did happen gradually. And pound by pound he gained weight.

Over the next few weeks, a lot of things went right and a lot of things went wrong. Back and forth. Eventually Pete started to realize that all this would come to an end and the harder he worked, the sooner things would improve. So he started walking more than once every day with his physical therapists, and eventually he was strong enough to walk with his walker and with me pulling his IV pole behind us. He started to compete with himself and try to do more laps every day. The old Pete was finally resurfacing. Pete has always appreciated his health and has never taken a day for granted.

We would walk so many laps every day around the 12th floor that I think we may have annoyed the nurses. They were constantly having to dodge Pete as he came shuffling around the corner. But he wasn't giving up.

Through all this recovery, Pete never once complained that he was now carrying a four-pound bag over his shoulder that he could never, ever get rid of. He seemed interested in learning more about it. He never showed any visible signs that he felt sorry for himself. He only seemed happy to be alive and was ready to adjust to his new situation.

Concurrently, I was being trained to take care of him. There was a lot of training that I was given regarding the VAD and it was a requirement. I also had to be shown how to change his bandage, which had to be done daily. Infection is the main cause of problems with VAD patients and much of that comes from infected incisions. The power cable runs from Pete's VAD controller in through an incision in his belly and up to the pump in his heart. That incision was what had to be cared for diligently. Sterile masks and gloves became my daily costume. I was determined to not let one single bad germ into Pete's body.

Things were progressing and now I had a new goal. To get Pete sprung from the hospital in time for his 50th birthday. It wasn't going to be easy because the days were ticking by. Pete would make progress then he would slip backward. He'd get stronger then he'd get an infection and a fever. It was a repetitive pattern.

At one point, we were so close to being released. Pete mentioned that he had a headache. I wouldn't have thought a thing about it. If I'd been the hospital for months, I imagine I would have had a headache too. But Greg Poulin, our wonderful nurse practioner, kept a super keen eye on Pete. He knew that there was no reason Pete should be suffering from a nagging headache.

He sent Pete for a CT scan and sure enough—bleeding on the brain.

We were so close to being released from the hospital, and all of a sudden it was back to ICU. This pattern seemed endless. Ups and downs. So like a flashback to the year before when Pete had had the stroke, I was again consulting with neurologists. Pete was watched closely over the next two days. Nobody could explain the bleeding. It could have been caused by the blood thinners. He wasn't showing any signs of a stroke, so that was encouraging. The doctor said it was very possible that the blood would slowly dissipate, and be absorbed back into his body.

During this stay, cousin Colleen came for the weekend to check in on both of us. She was there as we went back to ICU and was very comforting to us. Making him laugh and rubbing his swollen feet with lotion. At one point during the weekend, on June 11, Colleen disappeared into the waiting room to make a call. I noticed she'd been gone for quite a while. When I went out to check on her I could tell that something bad was happening. When she hung up, she looked at me and said that Tom, Pete's brother-in-law and T's husband, had died from a massive heart attack. He was a race walker and had collapsed and died instantly during a race earlier that morning.

It was a sad, sad day. Tom was a father figure to Pete. He had married Pete's sister when Pete was only nine years old. He looked up to him and credits him for creating his desire to be a musician. So how were we going to tell him? I was grateful that Colleen was with me. I was in over my head and not sure what to do. I actually pondered not telling Pete. I was so concerned about his fragile health. So I decided to check with his doctors to make sure it wouldn't cause more brain or heart trauma. After a short wait I got a call from the doctor on call that evening and he said it would be okay to give the news to Pete.

At the same time Colleen and I were in shock and wading through this dilemma, Pete was getting ready to Skype call his old high school friends in New Bern, NC. Les Wetherington, Mark Shelton and Cynthia Manning Martinez were throwing a huge benefit in his honor – a fundraiser to help us out with medical expenses. He was looking forward to it and I couldn't ruin his one moment of happiness with this horrible news. So we let him enjoy talking to his friends and listening to them perform for about 30 minutes while Cynthia walked around the New Bern celebration with a laptop allowing Pete to say hi to some old friends. Eventually he became so exhausted he told me he had to hang up. It was at that point that Colleen and I broke the news to him about Tom. He was surprised and saddened but not distraught. I don't think he had the energy to be distraught. He handled it well and was eventually able to talk to his sister on the phone. It was an unexpected event for everyone. Tom was well loved by everyone in his family and left a huge hole in all of us. That night Pete sat in his bed in ICU and composed a beautiful eulogy for Tom. He gave it to Colleen to read in his absence. He even asked her to rehearse it for him which was certainly a glimmer of the old Pete.

Pete's brain bleeding turned out to not to be a major problem. After about three days we were sent back to 12 Tower to work our way back to being released. Only 8 more days until Pete's 50th birthday. I knew he would be depressed if he had to celebrate this monumental birthday in a hospital.

He worked tirelessly getting his strength up so the doctors would feel he was well enough to be released into my care. He was eating a little bit better and continuing his incessant laps around the 12th floor.

After weeks and weeks of us not being at home, Sean was really starting to stress out. I wanted to come home, but every day in the hospital it looked like Pete could be discharged. I couldn't risk not being there when he was released. He would be sent "home" which in our case was an efficiency hotel room. I had to be there. So I couldn't plan any trips. I asked Sean if she wanted to come to Houston and she jumped at the chance. I wasn't sure if she'd be into it or not, but she was really looking forward to it.

She arrived two days before Pete's 50th birthday, and I think her visit there may have saved her mentally. I believe she was at her wits' end handling everything on her own. She was already anxiety ridden over leaving Liverpool and deciding where to go to school next. And she thrives on being a creature of habit. But with everything out of sync for so long, she really needed some support and it was impossible for me to go home and give it to her. So I flew her to us. The timing was perfect. She arrived on a Tuesday. She was so excited. I was excited and Pete was excited. We had discussed a few weeks earlier about flying the kids to Houston to see him, but we decided that he was just too sick, too sick looking and that instead of boosting their confidence that he'd be okay, it might have scared them even more. He truly looked like he was dying because he was so thin. And looking back on it, even though we decided the time was right for Sean to come, he still looked pretty terrifying, especially to your own stepchild. But he had improved so greatly in our mind, that we thought he looked fantastic. He did not.

So Sean was startled by his appearance, but was truly happy to see Pete. And I think his heart woke up when she walked into the room.

It felt like forever since we'd seen her. Her stress keeping things together back at home had hit a boiling point. She needed to see me, she needed to see Pete and she needed to get out of Nashville for a weekend. So she flew in and took a shuttle to the hotel. I was so happy. It was perfect timing because she would be able to help me get Pete from the hospital to our hotel/apart-ment. Texas Heart Institute was going to release him from the hospital, but not release him from Houston. He had to remain nearby for a couple of months in case he needed additional care, and it turns out he needed extensive care well after his release.

During our time in Houston, there were several volunteers that would visit with us in our hospital room. Miguel and Randy were the most visible. Miquel was also a VAD recipient and Randy was a heart transplant recipient who was celebrating his 20th year post transplant. They both came by the room on a weekly basis and shared so much joy.

Randy knew Pete's birthday was coming up. We'd been given the "go code" to leave the hospital on June 22, his 50th birthday. As much as we had worked toward this day, we were both a little bit freaked out. Pete procrastinated getting out of bed and getting dressed. It occurred to me that he wasn't in any hurry, but I couldn't figure out why. I went and found Peggy, our social worker. I told her something was up and that I thought Pete might be afraid to leave. She said it was a normal feeling and that she'd come and talk to him. Pete fessed up pretty quickly that he was very nervous. He didn't feel safe outside the hospital and he was afraid something would go wrong. She reassured him that the doctors wouldn't be releasing him if they didn't believe he was ready. He relaxed and started to let me help him get dressed.

Pete had a couple of surprises in store for his birthday. His good friend Jeff Taylor had sent Pete a ukulele for his birthday. He thought it would be easier for Pete to get his arms around than his guitar. Collings had the same idea and also sent a ukulele. They were both right and Pete was so pleased to have them. He still wasn't up to playing anything, but he enjoyed looking at them and holding them.

At that point, Randy walked into the room. He brought with

him a small birthday cake, candles, paper plates and forks. He said he knew that I didn't have a car and wouldn't be able to acquire all the necessities of a birthday celebration. I appreciated it so much. He was right. I never would have been able to pull it together.

Sean and I hurried to the hotel and compiled all the gifts Pete's family had sent including a huge bunch of balloons from his nieces, cards and letters, and now, a cake. We centered it all on a table right inside the door of the apartment. He couldn't miss them. Then we headed back to the hospital to get Pete.

There's a very special bell that hangs by the elevators at 12 Tower. The bell is for patients that have survived a heart transplant and are going home. Every now and then I'd hear that bell ring and I'd know that somebody had recovered enough to go back home to be with their families. Pete hadn't had a heart transplant. But I sure felt he'd earn the chance to ring that bell. So with Sean and me carrying everything that we'd accumulated over the course of two months on our shoulders and me with one hand on Pete, he rang that bell as we left the floor. I'd been waiting so long to hear that.

Chapter Thirteen

Support

Erin

As one who enjoys helping others, I have no idea why I'm not good at accepting help myself. I've thought about it and I still don't know if it's because I'm a control freak, stubborn, or just introverted. But I like to think I'm smart enough to know when I'm beaten and can't handle any more. So in Houston I turned myself over to the kindness and support of our family and friends. Pete's brother Frank put the word out to the Huttlinger clan, a large one, that I

153

was going to have to live in a hotel for several months. It was a call to action. Within days I received dozens of checks and had an entire month's hotel bill covered instantly. The wave of relief I felt was enormous. Especially since the narrative running through my mind was, "how will I survive if Pete never works again and I lose clients because I'm focused on taking care of Pete?" That type of conversation ran through my brain constantly – we had savings, but not enough to last years, let alone a lifetime. But getting my immediate needs covered quieted the voices in my head for a while and was a wonderful reprieve.

As the weeks rolled by I found financial support coming at me from all directions. It was such a foreign concept and my normal manner would have been to turn it all down. In fact, I had turned it down following Pete's stroke. But this time our future was looking pretty dire. There were so many possible scenarios. Pete could get right back to work and everything would be fine. That seemed like the least likely scenario. Or, Pete would survive but never be able to work again and my work would be limited because of his health. This was what I thought would be the most likely scenario. Or, Pete would not survive and there would still be a mountain of medical bills for me to have to handle. This was a scenario I just wouldn't consider.

But regardless, it was obvious even to me that I was going to need some sort of financial support for my family. I changed my outlook and was then able to truly appreciate all the checks that were being sent to us. MusiCares, an organization run by NARAS (National Association of Recording Arts and Sciences – popularly known for their Grammy Awards) reached out to us before we had even left Nashville for Houston. Over the course of those many months, MusiCares paid for all of our utility ex-

penses at home. They paid for the electric, gas, water, cable, etc…
the things we needed to keep the house running back in
Nashville. Fans from around the globe would take up a collection
and send us $1,000. Or someone that had very little themselves
would send us $5 with a beautiful letter or card saying how much
they loved Pete and hoped he would be well soon. The support
was amazing and I quickly learned that I needed it. Pete's income
really runs the household. He pays for our home and our cars and
utilities. He pays for all of our travels. My income covers a lot of
other things. But between the mortgage, his life insurance, health
insurance and utilities, that's a pretty big chunk of change each
month. And I also found that I didn't know what method he used
to pay all these bills. I had procrastinated for a couple of weeks,
but eventually put my mind to it, made a bunch of calls, and
thanks to some very, very helpful people at the bank, who had
known Pete for many years—they walked me through the bills,
the autopays and what came from what account. So every month
I knew exactly what needed to be covered and when. The
thought that I would accidentally not pay his health insurance
premium was so frightening that it kept me on my toes and I was
able to stay on top of most everything. But it was most definitely,
absolutely, because we had been given so much by so many.

But that's all about financial support. The emotional support
that I was offered can't have a dollar value attached.

I am so fortunate that my entire immediate family all live in
Nashville. My parents, Norma and Ed, my brother Jason and my
sister Rachel offered such wonderful emotional support. They all
volunteered to come to Houston and sit by my side, but I encouraged them to stay home in Nashville. I was okay. I wasn't fragile
anymore. The kind of support they gave me at home with the

kids gave me the mental freedom to not worry and to spend all my energies to keep Pete afloat.

Pete's side of the family is large in numbers and large of hearts. The contact was never broken. A family that has gone through countless tragedies is very inter-connected. There's a communication system that rivals that of the army. Phone trees got nothin' on these people. They can muster an Army of support within hours. Money, phone calls, care packages and visits were numerous and ongoing.

Pete was unaware of all the calls and flowers and messages, but they meant the world to me. Pete's niece Molly relieved me so I could go home to see the kids, his cousins Cath and Colleen came and spent time more than once and it was invaluable. In addition to lending a hand they could make me laugh and it felt good. My dear friend Marcy touched base with me every other day, sent me cookies and cards and offered to come to Houston. And my friend and business partner Alison Auerbach, along with my mother, covered my work and clients. I never felt like I was forgotten or that our dire situation was old news. Everyone kept it current for me and I learned a lot from that.

I would assume that most people don't know how loved they are until something goes wrong with their health and then folks are lined up to help and give support. I have to say that was only partially true in our case. Our families had been hugely supportive over the years, especially when we were on the road touring and needed an extra hand back at home with the kids. The same thing applies with fans. We have felt truly loved over the years as we would encounter friends as we travel and make new fans. And even with all the love and support, I never could have imagined how much additional support we would receive during Pete's health issues.

Over the years it had been my inclination to keep Pete's heart issues quiet. I was always concerned that it would impede his ability to tour successfully. As time went on, I would make some people aware of his condition, especially on those rare occasions when I couldn't be with him for a show. As certain incidents became more and more public, there was no option but to come clean and let his fans know what was going on. Especially since Pete has such a wicked sense of humor. He was very inclined to make jokes about his own health problems from the stage, whether it was the stroke or his heart problems. Slowly through this unveiling I also let people know that I was his wife as well as his manager. For his sake I had kept that under wraps, but my concern for his health was such an obvious tell that that bit of news became public as well.

As his manager I knew that it is truly alarming to fans to hear that their favorite performer is ill. And even though I gave myself a buffer of privacy and tried to make sure I was dealing with everything before I would share any details, I would eventually post information on Pete's Facebook and various social networking outlets including CaringBridge, which has been hugely helpful.

I would tend to write these updates late at night after everyone was asleep and I'd left the hospital and had a glass of wine. That fact that I was exhausted and tipsy probably made me a bit more forthcoming and less dry than I would have been otherwise. It seemed to work because fans and friends would write to me how much they really enjoyed the posts. In fact, they were on pins and needles if I didn't write often enough. In that case, no news was bad news to them. So even when I was exhausted I had to remind myself that everyone else in our universe was waiting for the most recent update.

But as much as it was helping me put into perspective the situation I was in by putting it into words, it also helped me cope and find a lot of joy. The responses I would get after each posting were amazing. The sheer quantity was difficult to grasp, but more than that it was the content.

Some messages were brief, some were lengthy. And it was gratifying to find out how deeply concerned people were, how it was consuming their thoughts. Every time I posted, I received dozens and dozens of thanks and admissions that they were worried since I had last written. There were responses from people that told how they'd never met us, never seen Pete perform. Yet a song, or one of the instructional videos had really changed their lives. And in some cases they really had changed their lives, or helped them heal after a health disaster. Many of these messages brought me to tears.

I would try to read them to Pete in the hospital but sometimes it was overwhelming. Partially due to the fact that it made him realize how sick he was and how people from around the world were watching his progress and communicating with us. It was something I could do with him when he was too sick to talk. I read to him sometimes and sometimes his brother Frank or cousin Cath would read these messages to him. But just a few at a time.

I have never experienced anything like this as far as mass support. Of course, I'd never needed it before either. Every single one of those people taught me something. And I was a good student. I have learned that people in dire straits aren't necessarily thinking clearly. Or perhaps they are but they are too exhausted to respond clearly, or to know what it is they need. I have learned that in order to help someone, just do it. It's okay to ask them specifically what they need, but if they don't know, just do it. Just fix something at the house, just take the kids out for dinner, just bring food even if you don't know what they like, just send money, bring groceries, weed the garden, take the dog for a walk. Just do something.

Chapter Fourteen

Now What?

Erin

Pete and I have an amazing connection. It's on a superficial level and it's on the deepest of levels. I believe that we are more one person than we are two. I would imagine a lot of couples feel that way. I can't hog that claim all to myself, but a lot of people comment that they wish they could have what we have. And Pete and I wish everyone could have what we have. It's outrageously wonderful and I can't imagine it any other way. If every couple were as connected and happy as we are, and always have been, then the world would be a different place.

I want to give you a picture, but I don't want to sound arrogant, braggadocios or unbelievable. But we really do feel the other's joy and the other's pain. We feel solitude and peace in the same way, we feel great depths of humor and it rattles throughout our bones—at the same time. It is my greatest hope that we can convey that connection to Sean and James and that they will look for a partner who can feel identically as excited about being with them as they do with the partner. It must be hard to find because so many people really don't have it. And if I knew how to make it happen I would be writing a book about that instead of about love and life and illness.

So, if one of us gets sick, the other one doesn't also get sick. But, the one who isn't sick compensates in an exactly parallel way to fill the void of the other. So again we are perfectly in tune. And that's what has happened over the last couple of years with Pete and me.

I can't feel directly what Pete is feeling physically or emotionally. I've never been in his shoes even remotely. But I can tell by the excruciating pain and stress I feel as I try to fill the void and compensate to keep the two of us in tune. In that way I can understand the enormity of what he is feeling. And as we are surrounded by so many wonderful doctors and family members and friends, I think I can say that they all feel their worry and pain in a certain way, but I feel it through Pete.

Pete and I have always worked in this way. He's the performer. I'm the manager. He's the on-stage comic. I'm the backstage comic. He's the driver. I'm the navigator. But even though we have our own roles, they have always meshed identically. The ebb and flow of our days, our nights, our years, and our lives stays perfectly in sync. When we first started working together he would call me "Radar" after Radar O'Reilly the adorable clerk on the TV series M*A*S*H. Radar would always bring the Captain what he needed just as he was asking for it. He had an uncanny knack for anticipating everyone's needs.

We have been able to handle any bad news we've received throughout our relationship because one had always been able to prop up the other. To be a true shoulder, and most importantly to help talk through whatever the situation calls for and come up with the best way to view it and, if it's a problem, to solve it.

The difference now was that I didn't have my sounding board. I didn't have that rational, loving partner to work with me. Pete was always able to tell me openly how he felt about his health and about whatever new predicament he was in. He could say, "I'm not worried about it," so then I wouldn't be worried about it. He could say that he was really disappointed in a doctor's visit and I'd help him find the positive angles of it. Or we might not understand the medical jargon we had just received, so we'd research it. Additionally, just with regards to doctor's appointments and medications, Pete has always been very involved and taken care of himself. I had never handed him a handful of pills or reminded him it was time to take them. He'd done it himself, his whole life.

Now he was in such a state that he couldn't take care of himself in any way at all. He could not even sit up on his own. He was 100% reliant on others to take care of him.

Often I needed to talk to him to tell me what the best decision was, but he wasn't there for me to access. It was the first time that I had to make choices without a safety net. I knew that I was capable and I trusted my own judgment, but life just wasn't as fun that way. In the worst situations we could still find humor. I could only think funny thoughts to myself. I probably could have shared everything that went through my head, which was the norm even when I'm sure he didn't want to know everything. But it would have been stressful for him. During his months of recovery, he really didn't have an opinion on anything. He didn't have a sense of humor at all. He didn't even laugh with his eyes. His day was all about survival into the next day.

I held back all the monotonous details of the day, and of all the household stuff going on back home. Even the littlest thing seemed to me to be too much data for him to endure. It would have zapped his only strength just to listen to me. But I did always reassure him that everything at home was fine and that the kids were in good shape.

I can't say that I felt lonely because I was always with him. And just being with him was a comfort. Just knowing that he was alive and improving, albeit slowly, gave me a mission. I never thought of myself as a wonderful mother or fabulous wife. Not in the traditional sense. Not in the stay-at-home mom way of doing things where every aspect of life revolves around the kids. And not in the perfect homemaker wife way of doing things that keeps a perfect house and makes perfect meals. But throughout this year I did realize that I had to pull every mother and wife skills out of my hat. Some that I didn't even know that I had. I had to problem solve in a brand new way and I think it worked. I guess I won't know until the kids are grown and Pete and I are old to find out if I did damage to anyone.

But now what? We were being released from the hospital. It was the same feeling I had when I brought Sean home from the hospital as a newborn. Now what? I've had a baby and all this build up has been terribly exciting, but now that part's over and I have to bring this fragile person home. How do I take care of her?

It was the same thing with Pete. All these weeks of trauma and recovery and now we had our freedom. Our opportunity to move back in the direction of our normal life. And I was terrified. I was now his nurse, his doctor, his social worker and his therapist. Just when I thought I had myself together, I realized that I was scared. What if he fell? What if he bled? What if the pump stopped working? I was a traumatized pile of nerves. And yet I was so excited to be in our own environment away from the hospital.

Sean helped me get Pete loaded onto the hospital shuttle that ran to our hotel. We were excited to sing "Happy Birthday" and share his presents with him. To this day, Sean and I laugh when we think about it. We got him to the apartment and threw open the door. There was the pile of gifts, balloons and cards. Pete didn't give them a second look. All he could see was the recliner across the room. He pushed his walker right past everything and asked me to help him into his chair. He was completely oblivious to the celebration. Sean and I looked at each other and just started smiling. Poor Pete felt so tired that he just wanted to sit down.

After a couple of days, Sean flew home to Nashville. Now it was just the two of us in the hotel. It only took a few days for me to acclimate. Initially we stuck to the same schedule as in the hospital, but with a more solid, less interrupted sleep schedule. Getting Pete to eat was still an issue. Mostly Cheerios, gingersnaps and milk. Then cousin Cath suggested Grape Nuts and yogurt. He really took to that. I fed him whatever he wanted whenever he wanted it and slowly he gained some weight.

Even though I had been in the hospital with Pete nearly all day, every day, I had not had to actually be his nurse. This was a little bit more stressful. If he fell, I was on my own. If something went awry with the heart pump, I was on my own. There were two double beds in the bedroom. Pete slept in one and I slept in the other. He was so fragile still that I didn't want to accidentally bump him in the middle of the night or make him uncomfortable in any way. He was so weak and had been hospitalized for so long. Throughout the night, every couple of hours or so, he would wake up and need help shifting his position or need to go to the bathroom. I would help him with both.

One afternoon when he awoke from a nap, he called me over to the bed. He asked me to help him roll over. It wasn't that he didn't have the strength now to roll over—he just couldn't re-member how to do it. It was the strangest thing and it was an-other one of the moments where we both realized just how screwed up things had gotten. He could not remember what mus-cles to use, and in what order, to get from his back over to his side. So I went through those basic steps in my mind and told him to move his arm this way, his hip that way, use his knee to pull himself over to one side. He was so appreciative and then we both just kind of laughed at the situation.

Getting himself dressed and cleaned up every day was a slow ordeal as well. He would sit on his walker with his head over the bathroom sink and I'd wash his hair. As long as he was stable, I encouraged him to dress himself as much as he could. Shoes and socks were out of the question though. He couldn't make that reach, so I would do that part for him.

Pete enjoyed being out of the hospital. Every day, we would

walk the halls of the hotel for exercise. We'd walk down the carpeted hallway until we reached the end, touch the wall, then turn
and walk back. Over and over again. For a while we did it with his
walker, and eventually without the walker. His gait was very un-
steady so I tried to stay right beside him in case he needed me to
catch him. He stumbled a lot, partly due to weakness and partly
due to the fact that his right side was still weak from the stroke.
He tended to not pick up his right foot (that continues to be an
issue today), causing him to trip.

Throughout the two months we lived in the hotel together, he
was probably in the hospital more than he was in the hotel. He
would get a fever and be readmitted. His blood work would be
out of balance and he'd be readmitted. His blood levels would get
too low and he'd be readmitted for transfusions. It was ongoing,
and every time he had to go back he would look at me with this
"I'm gonna' kill you for bringing me back here," look on his face.
I felt so guilty, but I learned to disregard it.

Once, when we were walking into the hospital from the parking garage for a doctor's appointment, he tripped on a curb and
fell flat on his face. He was bleeding, but conscious. He couldn't
get up. I finally helped him to his knees. Even at a low 120
pounds, dead weight isn't easy to move. He had blood on his face.
The irony occurred to me that I was actually already at the hospital so I couldn't call 911. I was certain he'd broken his nose. His
face was dripping blood because his sunglasses had cut into his
forehead. I had nothing to stop the bleeding. I saw a woman getting into her car in the parking garage. She had a baby in a
stroller. DIAPERS! They're absorbent. I ran to her and asked for
a small disposable diaper which she quickly handed me. Pete held
that to his forehead and we walked the 100 yards to St. Luke's

ER. My heart was pounding and nerves were shot. But even in these moments we could find things to laugh about. Since Pete's glasses had embedded into his face, and because he was on blood thinners, the nurses wouldn't try to remove the glasses until the doctor could see him—afraid he might bleed more. So he sat there in his ER room, on the table with his sunglasses on the whole time. I teased him that he was acting like a rock star. They eventually stitched him up and sent us back home.

Pete

Two times a week, a fellow named Hector would come to our hotel to work me through rehabilitation exercises. This was the most basic kind of rehab, which included walking on a flat surface, going upstairs, and building muscle in my arms and legs. I'm sure I was not the most exciting patient he'd dealt with and actually I dreaded each and every one of his visits. I would stay in bed too long, trying to act like I was still asleep. Erin would wake me and remind me that Hector was coming. I needed no reminding. I just didn't want to participate.

But he'd show up with his scale, several bungee type cords and sheets of paper for us to fill out. He would weigh me first. 125 pounds was a number I just couldn't get above. I was eating a little more than I had been eating at the hospital, but not much. Part of the problem was that everything tasted like dirt. All the meds I'd had for so long messed with my taste buds. The nurses gave me the go ahead to eat anything I wanted, no holds barred. Just eat. But who wants to eat dirt? Not me. So 125 pounds was the best I could do for him.

Hector started out walking with me down the hallway at the hotel. The floors were all carpeted and I would occasionally trip wherever the carpet had buckled. It was an Extended Stay after all not the Four Seasons so the carpet was a little iffy. When we first began he would put his arm around me to steady me while we walked. Up and down the hallway two times was it for me. I was pretty tired.

Then back into our room and out came the bungee cords. He would wrap one end around the doorknob then put the other end around my leg, low near my foot. I'd stand with a chair to balance myself and pull back with my leg. I really felt like I was wimping out but 6 or 7 times with each leg and I'd be done. It was hard and really, who wants to do something that's hard? Not me and not then.

Now for the arms. Hector would leave the bungee's on the doorknob and I'd pull on them with my arms. Sometimes like a pull-up motion and other times I'd have to put my arms straight by my side. Then pull straight back.

"C'mon Pete, pull harder," Hector would say.

"I'm pulling, I'm pulling," I'd reply exasperated.

"You are? I think the bungee should be moving if you're pulling."

Sometimes we'd go out of the room to the stairwell. The dreaded stairwell! God how I hated this part. I knew I needed it but I was certain that Hector and the devil were in cahoots on this one. We started with two steps.

"C'mon Pete, give me two. You can do it."

"I don't know Hector. That seems like a long way from here. How about if we just start with one?"

"Okay, we'll start with one… then we'll just add one more."

"That sounds suspiciously like two to me, Hector."

The first time he came I gave Hector those two steps. I liked down a whole lot more than up. Down was easier. Most of the time when I was still in the hospital I managed to weasel my way out of doing stairs. I could do all of the laps on the floor but there were no stairs involved. My therapist at the hospital, Kristen, didn't make me do them very often.

Turning around on the step involved a somewhat lengthy process. I had to lift my right leg over the step above, turn my body to the left (this was the hardest part since all of my weight was now on one leg), put my right foot back on the step, switch hands on the railing, steady myself then I could walk down. Something we all take for granted was so hard.

Back into the room Hector would have me lie down on the bed. Then with both legs straight out in front of me, lift one leg up as far as I could and hold it.

"Pete, I said hold it."

"I did hold it, Hector."

"How long would you say you held your leg up?"

"Seemed like about a minute to me."

"It was five seconds. Try it again."

I couldn't pull anything over on Hector. I really liked him but I dreaded his arrival. In between his visits to our hotel Erin would encourage me to work out. Sometimes I would but not always. We did, however, start walking down the steps from our floor instead of taking the elevator. Then we would walk up a flight to get back to our room. I remember feeling a real sense of accomplishment each time I would walk up a flight of stairs. Inside I knew that I was getting stronger, albeit slowly.

Erin and I had timed ourselves at the hospital when we walked laps. Fourteen laps equaled one mile. It would take about 30 minutes. So at the hotel we would walk up and down the hallway, touching the wall at each end each time. Sometimes for twenty minutes. Sometimes for thirty. I knew we were getting somewhere when we'd walk in the morning and then again in the evening. Slowly but surely I was regaining my strength.

Erin

Now it was time. I'd been waiting patiently. It was time to pull out God's Guitar — his favorite Collings OM-1. I had brought it back from Nashville after my last trip home to check on the kids. He has such a strong connection to that guitar; I assumed it would overcome any illness.

In the hotel room, Pete spent his time either sleeping or moving from the couch to the recliner. Anywhere his bony body could feel comfortable. One day while he was sitting on the couch, I pulled the guitar out and leaned it up near where he was sitting. He just let it sit there for a while. Eventually he picked it up, strummed it a couple of minutes and then put it down and ignored it. I could tell he was frustrated. The next day I did the same thing. He picked it up, strummed it and talked about how he wasn't going to play anymore. I just ignored him and continued to repeat the pattern. Each time I could tell that it bothered him that he couldn't play and I'd get sad when he would say that he'd never play again, or that he'd learn to do something different. But I knew in my heart that Pete and that guitar were one. That he didn't just want to play, he had to play it. I also knew that I would be heartbroken if I could never hear him make music again. I couldn't accept it. Then slowly but surely he started to ask me to hand him his guitar. I knew he was headed in a positive direction.

Meanwhile, back in Nashville, another benefit was being

planned. Some of our friends in the industry – Bob Burwell and Neal Spielberg – put together a great concert lineup and the Mercy Lounge donated the space. The benefit was scheduled for July 26. It was highly unlikely that Dr. Bogaev was going to release us from her care in time. But, we made a deal. If she'd let us fly home for Sean's 19th birthday on July 25 and the benefit on July 26, we'd come right back to Houston. She agreed and we started getting excited about making a visit home.

Chapter Fifteen

The Benefit

Pete

One of the greatest things about Nashville is the sense of community that resides there. People reaching out to help others. Almost every week there is a benefit concert for someone. Someone who has cancer or someone whose husband passed away unexpectedly. Someone who has a sick child or someone who lost everything in a fire or flood. Folks come out and play music. And others come out and listen. I don't know which comes first: the

173

love of music or the desire to help those in need. But they are always there hand in hand.

Bob Burwell and Neal Spielberg, along with our friend Jason Henke, told Erin of their plans to host a benefit concert for us. They would have Scott Goldman, who is the Vice-President at the Grammy Foundation, host the entire event. (The Grammy Foundation was established to cultivate the understanding, appreciation and advancement of the contribution of recorded music to American culture.) Erin was very uncomfortable being the recipient of such an endeavor but she knew enough to know that we were going to be out of work for a long time and we would need all the help we could get. After years of living in Nashville, both Erin and I had attended many benefit concerts. We had worked on them for people neither of us knew and for those whom we did know. It's that sense of giving that we both thrive on. So she accepted. But she said that she would not be able to help with it since she was in Houston taking care of me. Erin is a music industry publicist and normally that is when she kicks into high gear - when it is time to get the word out. They told her not to worry.

I was released from captivity in Houston on a five-day furlough to go home for Sean's 19th birthday and the benefit concert. But I would have to return immediately after the concert. So we flew from Houston to Nashville. That in itself was quite an experience. Learning to travel with a VAD, a bag full of medicines and a suitcase full of batteries was going to take some getting used to.

I remember going through security at Houston-Hobby airport and thinking "They're going to tackle me or shoot me because I have a bag hanging over my shoulder with wires coming out of it that go up under my shirt." I looked like an Auschwitz-styled terrorist. Skinny as skinny could be at 125 lbs. Clothes that didn't fit. And I was hard-wired for business. Yup, I was a goner for sure.

But as luck would have it, we were not the first to go through the airport with a VAD. In fact, they had a special line at security which was designated MEDICAL LINE. They must have known we were coming and put in a special line just for us. Our good friends Kevin and Pat Stewart picked us up at the airport in Nashville. It was great to see them. They didn't expect to see me walking. Mission accomplished.

We were so excited to be home again after three months. It was only for five days but what a fantastic break it was from Houston. We got to sleep in our bed, eat at our dining room table. Watch our TV. Yes, it's the little things in life that made us feel so comfortable and relaxed.

We knew that Vince Gill was going to be there to perform. So would Buddy Green and Jeff Taylor. John Jorgensen, my step-daughter Sean Della Croce, Sam Bush, Brent Anderson, Cynthia Manning Martinez, John Oates, Kathie Baillie, Michael Bonagura, Alyssa Bonagura, Bekka Bramlett, Mark Selby, Bill Lloyd, The Long Players, Chuck Fields and many others. They all offered their amazing talents to the concert. Jeff Hanna from The Nitty Gritty Dirt Band called Erin and left her a message. He'd heard about the benefit and wanted to perform if there was a spot open for a vocalist. She was thrilled. She saved his message on her phone.

I remember how sick I felt the day of the benefit. Normally I would sleep a good part of the day. I would get up, eat and then nap for an hour or two after breakfast. Nap for an hour or two after lunch. And then ten to twelve hours at night as well. But being at home I was excited to see friends and I was not getting the rest I was used to.

When we arrived at the Mercy Lounge in Nashville, there was a long line outside and I was thrilled that so many folks would show up. The first people I spotted in line were our friends Charlie and Barbara White from Florida. They came all that way and I was touched. It was the first of many times that day I would feel so moved.

July 26, 2011 was a long day. We thought we might go to the concert for a little while and then head home. But when we arrived and I saw so many friends and acquaintances, I just couldn't leave. Erin asked me earlier in the day if I wanted to play a song with John Oates of Hall & Oates. John had become a very good friend over the years and I really wanted to do it. But I knew that I couldn't play the guitar very well at all. I made a beginner look like Segovia that day. I could barely hold on to a flat-pick let alone a guitar. But at the last moment I agreed to do it.

I recall walking up the steps to the stage and legendary bluegrass artist Sam Bush was standing there and he asked if I needed help. I told him yes. At that time I was able to walk up about five steps in our hotel work-outs and then I would head back down. That was it. I was shocked at how many steps were there at The Mercy Lounge — just to get to the stage. There were fifteen by my count on that night. So Sam helped me up the steps, John Oates introduced me and a very understanding audience gave me a round of applause as I stumbled my way through an arrangement I had originally arranged for John of John Denver's song Leaving On A Jet Plane. I knew that he was going to ask me about playing that song so I had looked it over earlier in the day. But in typical artist fashion John turned to me and said, "I've changed a few things in this one Pete. Just follow me," and then he immediately started the tune. Now normally that would not be a problem for me. I'm used to last minute changes. But on this day I could barely play the guitar, much less follow someone through a Philly-style arrangement of this song. So at times I just stood there and listened to him. Then when I knew what was coming I would play along. It was a disastrous performance and a beautiful moment that I will never forget as long as I live.

My step-daughter Sean walked on stage for her performance. She told the audience some beautiful things about how I had influenced her musically. Then she did a fantastic performance of the Johnny Cash song "Folsom Prison Blues." She had a great young guitarist named Joe Robinson lined up to play with her but he contacted someone the night before saying that he was stuck in Rome, Italy and would not be able to make the show. So Erin and Sean hemmed and hawed about what to do. I don't recall if it was me or Erin but one of us suggested we ask Vince Gill to play guitar with Sean on the Johnny Cash tune. He was scheduled to be there and perform anyway and I know how much he loves to play the guitar...almost as much as me. Vince agreed without a second thought. Their performance was the highlight of the evening for me. Seeing my step-daughter up on the stage with Vince accompanying her and the look on Vince's face when Sean was singing a high G note at the end was priceless.

Someone asked me if I would do a brief interview backstage with Vince for "Headline Country" a national entertainment tv show. I said sure thinking 'they don't know how sick I really am, do they?' So Erin led me to the backstage area and I found Vince and the camera guy along with show host Storme Warren who was going to conduct the interview. As I recall it went something like this:

Storme – "Vince, tell us a little bit about Pete and this concert."

Vince – "Well, Pete's a really fine player and we're all out here to help him and his lovely wife Erin…" He continued on for a few minutes…

Storme – "Pete, do you have anything to add to that?"

Me – "Nope," I said with little enthusiasm. It was late and I was sick and I was tired.

Storme – "Vince, so Pete has a heart pump. What do you know about that?"

Vince – "Yes, he does. We're all so happy for Pete and Erin…" He continued on for a few minutes being the pro that he is.

Storme – "Pete is there anything, anything at all that you'd like to add to what Vince has already told us."

Me – "Nope."

It was late and I was sick and I was tired. I could barely stand and I doubt that the interview ever made it to air.

My sister, T, was there as well. She looked shell-shocked from her husband Tom's death. Her best friend, lover, reading, drinking, child-raising, traveling and camping buddy for the past forty years had died.

On top of that, her baby brother looked like a scarecrow and most of the folks who attended that night hadn't seen me in forty pounds or so, so many of them thought I was a goner. I can only imagine what she must have thought when she saw me. Several of the attendees told me, after I got healthier, that they thought that was the last time they'd see me.

But T made the best of it. She sat with us for a long time.

Then as the night went on longer and longer, she stood up near the stage. I remember when Vince, Jeff Hanna and Jim Hoke were playing the old Nitty Gritty Dirt Band hit, Mr. Bojangles. I watched my sister and knew that she'd be okay. There was a spark in her as she swayed back and forth to the music and it was a beautiful thing to see. I wish I'd have had the strength to tell her that night that things would be okay for her.

My good friend of many years, Jeff Cox, came by our table. I thought I must have looked like death to him but he merely smiled, patted me on the back and said how good it was to see me.

My old pal, Steve Emley was there as well. Making sure that I had everything I needed. I think the only request I had was for some ice-water. I mentioned it to Steve and it magically appeared. Steve was good at keeping people from cr owding me too. He has worked for several years as a tour manager for many music artists and he's very good at what he does. I don't like denying access to people but this night was different. I was sick and could only talk for a minute to a select few.

Erin's brother Jason, her sister Rachel with her husband Jody and their kids, her mom and dad, and her cousins Leah and Marnie were all there as well.

And there were doctors. Lots of doctors, and nurses, and nurse practitioners. Ones who had taken care of me after the stroke and ones who had taken care of me through all my heart issues.

To say that the love in the room was palpable that night would be the understatement of this entire book. I have never felt so much good will and kindness from so many people in my life as I did that night. When I concentrate, I can still feel it from time to time. I wasn't able to walk around in the crowd or really even talk to many people. Erin, however, was able to walk through the crowd a time or two and told me that she saw so many wonderful friends from over the years, and was surprised to see so many of the Vanderbilt doctors and nurses that have cared for me.

At one point John Oates started an auction for a pair of tickets to a Hall & Oates concert. At first the bidding was slow and I was worried for John but then all of a sudden the price started going up and up and up. It turned into two pairs of tickets to a Hall & Oates concert anywhere in the world with backstage passes and he even offered up Daryl's wine from his dressing room as a joke.

The Hall & Oates tickets were auctioned off for over $7,000 total! Oh my God! I was stunned. With all the money from the ticket sales for the concert, that total put us at over $12,000! I was shocked to say the least. The manager at The Mercy Lounge did the unthinkable that night when he even gave up the club's commission from the ticket sales! He said that the take at the bar was so good that he was happy to contribute all the money directly to Erin and me.

I was back at Mercy Lounge in the fall of 2012 playing at a benefit concert hosted by Lance Hoppen of Orleans to help his relatives since his brother's passing. Those fifteen steps that Sam Bush helped me up…? There were only THREE of them. I could have sworn that there were fifteen. I remember looking up at the stage on the night of my benefit concert and it seemed so very far away.

Chapter Sixteen

The Shift In Pete

Erin

After the benefit we were bummed about having to come back to Houston. It was so good to be home if only briefly. But I think Pete went back with a determination to get better and to return to Nashville permanently.

During our entire time in Houston, we continued to have ongoing conversations with some of the doctors at Vanderbilt University Medical Center. Even though Texas Heart Institute ruled out a transplant, Vanderbilt did not. So we still continued to believe that Pete's VAD, in the end, wouldn't be a permanent thing. That we would get him healed and strong, that his lung pressures would improve and that Vanderbilt would do a transplant. We locked in great hope for that.

Still, Pete never complained about his new device. We tried different methods of carrying it around. Over his shoulder, in a backpack, different sized bags. Ultimately, the design that Heart-Ware had created for it seemed to work the best.

As Pete continued to gain strength in the hotel, he began to meet more people in his situation. He would have clinic appointments weekly and there he ran into a waiting room full of people with VADs. One smiling and rotund gentleman with a VAD came up to Pete to talk. He could tell Pete was a newer patient. Pete expressed his concern that he wasn't able to eat or put on weight. The man patted his own huge belly and told Pete not to worry, that he'd bulk up soon. I saw the look on Pete's face and knew that he hoped he wouldn't bulk up quite that much.

Ironically, Pete spent the last two weeks before we returned to Nashville back in the hospital. They had determined that an ongoing infection in him was attached to one of the devices in his chest, either the heart pump or the pacemaker. The only way to get rid of it was to replace them and obviously that wasn't an option anybody was interested in.

Pete

Two weeks before I was released from Texas Heart Institute a change came over me. I went from Pete the guy who is so sick and can't do anything for himself to Pete, the guy who can encourage others to get up and walk! Just like I had been encouraged by patients at the hospital, it was now my turn to lend a few words of support to others.

I had been readmitted to Texas Heart Institute for another week or so for an infection that was attached to either my VAD or my pacemaker/defibrillator. The docs were scratching their heads trying to figure out how to get rid of this doggone infection.

While I was there, Erin brought my little classical guitar in for me to try and play. I was trying but that was really about all I could do. Try. I was just a skeleton of my old self and as a player I was simply not a competitor. I had doubts whether I would ever perform again. I had to play the classical guitar because my normal choice, my Collings OM1, was too difficult to play. It hurt to press the strings down. I mean it hurt! I thought to myself why in the world would someone go through all this pain to play? It couldn't have hurt this much the first time I learned the guitar

My head remembered everything I was supposed to be able to do but my hands just couldn't do it. I would try to play a tune, any tune and it was disastrous. So I suggested to Erin that we learn some old songs that we could sing together. She has a great ear for music and she agreed. So we learned a few songs together. Then a nurse came in to the room and she said, "I didn't know you played the guitar. Hey, I've got a patient who is feeling kind of down. Would you come and play for him? He says he's a guitar player too." If he was in the same boat as I was, he couldn't be much of a player anymore, I thought to myself. But there was something in me that got excited to go and play for someone so I agreed. I got up slowly, grabbed my guitar.

I arrived, said hello and asked the young man if he wanted me to play a tune for him. He was not in a good mood at all but he said okay. So I sat down and I played the one thing I knew I could get through: "Lucky Southern" by Keith Jarrett. It's a simple Latin-flavored tune and it was an okay performance. Then the guy came to life and started asking me questions about my guitar and my background. "I used to be a player but not anymore," I told him. "Keep it up. You'll get it back," he replied.

Now after a couple of tunes in his room another nurse came by and looked at me and said, "When did you start playing the guitar? I didn't know you played that thing. Hey will you come and play for my patient? He's not feeling too good today." So off I went to another room, IV pole in one hand and guitar in the other to play a few tunes for someone else.

The next thing I knew I was on the circuit. I had the gig at 12 Tower of St. Luke's Episcopal Hospital playing for the patients. This was the best gig of my life in my opinion. I had been transformed from someone who was a sick patient to someone who was helping others heal. I was still very sick. I weighed in at around 125 lbs. I was a shadow of my old self. But I could walk a miles' worth of laps around the hospital floor now and I was eating a little more each day.

One of the nurses said that George Strait was her favorite singer and "Amarillo By Morning" was her favorite song. I would sing that song for her on every shift. I walked out of my room to the nurses' station and played for them all. They seemed so appreciative.

This was when my attitude changed. This was when everything started to turn around for me.

I was finally able to give something back to others and that is what makes me feel best. I could stop focusing on me for a little while each day and focus on another patient who was worse off than I. That was when I told Erin that I had a goal of leaving Houston in one week. I had a goal and she was excited.

That night I phoned our friend Jim Curry in California and spoke to him for an hour! I hadn't spoken to anyone for more than a few minutes (usually just a few seconds) for over five months and I had just spent an entire hour on the phone with Jim. We talked about music and his CD that we were going to do together. I couldn't believe it. I was actually making plans. I didn't tell him that I could not play well enough to record anything. I figured I would be well enough when the time came.

Then I called my cousin Cath in Massachusetts and I spent another hour on the phone with her. What a day that was. I told her all about my day at the hospital and about my new gig. I was fairly confident with my standing in the new gig, I told her, since no one ever came up to 12 Tower to play music for patients there. We were all too sick! No one would be allowed up there to play for us. But I had an "in." I was one of them and the gig was mine. Talk about a captive audience!

Erin

I don't know exactly what happened that day, but I can tell you a switch flipped in Pete's brain. When he came back to his hospital room where I was waiting, he was a different man. He changed over the course of 30 minutes. He was smiling bigger than he had in months. He was talkative. My old Pete was back!

Chapter Seventeen

"Lean On Me, Pete"

Pete

Everyone needs a champion when they are going through hard times and all through my health struggles, Erin has been mine. She didn't just sit in the waiting room during my surgery, she didn't just go to a few meetings with the cardiologists or the transplant team, and she didn't just take a few notes about my medicine regimen. Erin was there for each and every meeting with each doctor, nurse

187

practitioner, and nurse. When I was in the hospital, she met them first thing in the morning and was there to say goodnight to them when they went home for the night. She always took detailed notes and kept a notebook with her where she would write lots of questions to ask the doctors when they returned.

Erin is good with information. She would disagree with me on this but she has a great capacity for remembering large quantities of data and regurgitating it all verbatim weeks, months, even years later. She takes detailed notes and when she sees something that doesn't add up, she speaks up. A doctor's worst nightmare can be a patient's best friend. What a friend I have in Erin.

Erin is also very smart in the way she deals with people. I tend to shoot from the hip and it usually gets me in hot water. Not her. No. She will analyze a situation, ponder it in her mind and decide on a course of action that will usually assure that she gets what she needs and that you get what you need as well.

But her main focus throughout my illness was me, Pete. She wanted me to be healthy again. I have been very blessed in my life in many ways. Professionally I have achieved things I didn't even bother dreaming of because they were too far off my radar. I never would have thought I'd be performing at Carnegie Hall three times or at the first three of Eric Clapton's Crossroads Festivals but I did. I didn't think I would be at the famed Abby Road Studios recording with LeAnn Rimes but I was. I never thought I would be in London's Royal Albert Hall, or perform with the Houston Symphony, or travel to Vietnam, South Korea, Malaysia, Singapore, Ireland, Scotland, Australia, Hawaii, all with John Denver but I did that, too, and lots more.

Personally I have struggled with relationships. My home life as a child was as dysfunctional as one could imagine. (Mostly I remember lots of fist fights between my brothers. Not the kind where someone apologizes afterwards but the kind where they merely take a break for dinner and then continue to pummel the shit out of each other immediately afterwards. Occasionally, I was the receiver of such attention.) My first marriage had failed after 20 years. Because my dad died when I was three and my mom never remarried, I had no training in a good relationship but when I met Erin, everything fell into place.

She was nice to me. She listened to me and seemed interested in things I had to say. And I loved to hear her talk. We still can sit and talk for hours on end and this is after we've worked together for fifteen years and have been married for over eight.

She enjoys it when I play my guitar – sometimes for hours on end. Sometimes the same thing over and over and over again. She smiles and says it sounds good to her. The day we married, we had friends at our home playing music together for nearly eight hours. In my previous marriage I doubt that there was a combined total of "jamming" of eight hours in our house for the twenty years we were married. At one point Erin hiked up her wedding dress and played her hammer-dulcimer and the crowd at our wedding cheered her on.

I suggested we learn how to cook – really good food - and we did. I suggested we learn a foreign language and while we can't converse in it, we can order food and wine, find a hotel and offer our compliments when we travel to Italy. That's good enough for me.

Always ready for an adventure, Erin is the perfect match for me. We are each strong on our own but we are stronger together. Which brings me to my point for this section: Erin is more than my better half. She truly is the wholeness and completeness of me. We spend nearly every waking moment together not because we have to but because we enjoy each other's company that much.

I would not be alive today if it were not for Erin. It really is that simple and I really do believe it. She was with me almost every day in the hospital. She took great care of me in our little hotel room in Houston. Getting up every night when I would have to use the bathroom to help me out of bed and back into it. Before I could shower, she would dip my head in the little sink and wash my hair. As I regained my strength she would (and still does) put saran wrap over the bandage that covers the wires that come out of me so I could climb into the shower. She then changed the bandages after I got out. On Sundays she doled out my medicine for the week.

Erin never once complained about her struggles in taking care of me. How could she not? I can't say that I'd have been able to do the same, but she never did.

I could never say it properly in a book. But I love Erin. That's all.

I had been in the hospital for the biggest part of the past five months. The last time Erin and I made love was in mid-March 2011 in Charleston, West Virginia. It was the end of our road trip and we would be heading home. I was not feeling so good but we were both willing.

Now fast forward to five and a half months later. I felt bad for Erin because I knew what she had been going through for so long taking care of me, worrying about me, taking on all the bills, dealing with doctors, living in another city, missing her kids and the rest of her family. But I only knew that on a cerebral level. I had nothing in my life to relate to what she had been doing. I was always the receiver of such goodness and care.

I know how important the human touch is to all of us and she was getting none of that. I had no strength to speak of and I was a whopping 125 pounds. Gaunt, drawn out. But one Saturday night a week before I was released from Houston, I gave her the eye. She said "No way. We've gotten this far and I'm not going to be the one to kill you." I suggested that we may be able to make it happen so that I'm not so exhausted. I let it rest at that as she thought about it.

Later that night we made tender love and I knew then that it was the right thing to do not just for Erin but for both of us. Sex is such a wonderful way of releasing everything that builds up inside of us. While it may not go on forever, the good that it does for us lasts for several days at a time.

It's interesting that of all the patients I've encouraged over the years not once has the subject of sex ever come up. I've spoken to folks who were pondering heart pumps and some still in the hospital and many who've been released. No one has ever asked, "Can I still have sex if I have a heart pump?" Well, for those who are wondering but are afraid to ask the answer is a resounding, "Yes!" And it's still as great as it was before.

Erin

All I can say on this subject is that I had resigned myself to the fact that Pete and I would probably never again have sex. I couldn't imagine him ever being back to his original self. I didn't like it, but in the big picture it didn't affect how much I loved him. When he surprised me with the eye, I was hesitant to say the least. He was so fragile I was certain he would just shatter. I thought of how I was going to have to explain it to everyone if I ended up killing him after all the work we'd put into keeping him alive. But the good news is, I didn't kill him.

Chapter Eighteen

Leaving Houston

Erin

After almost exactly four months in Houston, Texas
we were released from the Care of the Texas Heart
Institute and returned to the care of Vanderbilt
University Medical Center.

Texas Heart Institute would continue to see us every six
months in addition to all the regular care at Vanderbilt. The ongoing care from Texas Heart Institute was based on the fact that
Pete was given "compassionate use" approval of the heart pump

since it was not officially FDA approved at the time, and also he wasn't part of the original study. Because of that, we had an obligation to be seen by them twice a year so they could keep accurate data on Pete's progress. This was not any problem to us because we had established a great comfort level and trust with all the doctors there. In fact, Vanderbilt was still not implanting the HeartWare device and wouldn't be until FDA approval was granted. There was a lot of politics, government red tape and finagling to make sure that Vanderbilt would have the computers and data they needed to resume Pete's care in Nashville, so we could be at home, finally.

We would think we were so close to getting released, then something would happen, Pete would get a fever, or need a transfusion. A recurring infection was just ruthless and every time we'd think it had been killed, it would return. And that was what was keeping us held in Houston most intensely, near the end of our stay. After weeks of battling the infection Pete was almost given the all clear. He'd been disappointed so many times that he was feeling pretty defeated and we both felt like we'd never get home. Pete had been back in the hotel room with me for a week or so. On Friday he'd given his blood for testing and we were supposed to get word on Monday. If the results were good, then they would release us. Pete was so anxious that he wouldn't get out of bed. He literally stayed in bed until almost noon with the covers over his head. He just couldn't take any more bad news. Finally, he asked me to call Dr. Kielhofner's office and get the results. It was good news. We were both so happy. Pete called Dr. Bogaev's office and reported that we'd been given the all clear from Dr. Kielhofner….and could we go home? The nurse said "yes." It seemed too easy. Do we need to come and see anyone? Get any papers?

Sign anything? The nurse basically told us that if it were him, he'd just hightail it out of town. So that's what we did.

But it couldn't happen fast enough for Pete. I'd been dug into our hotel apartment since late April. I had stuff to pack. Pete couldn't help me do any of it. All he could do was sit and look worried that they'd revoke our pass out of town. So he stared at me while I packed as fast as I could. We gave food away to other patients' families in the hotel. I threw away and boxed up at a frenzied pace. Then Pete monitored me as I packed the car. I felt for him, but I felt for myself, too. It was kind of hysterical. I was sweating in 103 degree weather. Late August in Houston. There's nothing like it. And my nerves were frayed because I knew Pete would be crushed if they recalled him for any reason. I couldn't let him down but I couldn't go any faster.

After a couple of hours of intense labor, the car was packed with all our belongings including a guitar and two ukuleles, all our clothes, medical supplies, gifts, computers, and us.

Of course, Pete couldn't drive either, so I'm in the driver's seat ready for a long two-day trip back home. On August 22, 2011, we left Houston just as rush hour was warming up. Pete was so happy and I knew I would be once we got on the open road. Then my phone rang. It was the hospital. We recognized the number. Pete answered it and one of the LVAD coordinators was on the line saying that we needed to sign some papers. "Too late," Pete told her. "We are already gone. You can fax them to our house in two days, and we promise we'll send them right back to you. But we aren't turning this car around." And we didn't.

Pete Huttlinger and Erin Morris Huttlinger

Chapter Nineteen

Back Home

Erin

It was so wonderful to be back in Nashville. I definitely felt like I was flying without a net, but I was ready. And actually that wasn't true – there was a net. There were constant appointments with Pete's doctors at Vanderbilt. They had stayed pretty closely tuned in to what was going on in Houston. Quite a number of the doctors had changed, but they were still aware of Pete's case.

I was so happy to be with my family again. The kids especially. Sean was just getting ready to start school at Belmont University (Nashville). We made it home the night before her first day. It felt so normal to be there to see her off. And poor James had registered himself for his junior year at Father Ryan High School. It certainly wasn't the way I envisioned starting their school year, but it was the way it was and I knew enough to not lament that lost time very much.

But I sure did try to make it up to them as much as I could. So did Pete. Even as sick as he was he would bundle up and I would drive us both on Friday nights to see James march in the band at football games. We would arrive just before half-time and stay not much past that. That was all that Pete had strength for. But we were there and it made James smile that huge smile that he has.

It was a brief period of readjustment. I had lived a very secluded life for four months. And now I was back at home with the all the things that go along with that. Everyday things. Less traumatic things.

In some ways I became so accustomed to handling things on my own that after months and months, as Pete slowly became able to do certain things for himself, I had to retrain myself again. I had to slowly turn things back over to him. Sometimes I knew he couldn't do it and even though he insisted I stood at the ready to take over. And sure enough I was right. I didn't feel good being right, and I'm sure it added to his humiliation over being so helpless, but it was what it was. But sometimes he was ready to take over a task for himself. And it was a beautiful thing. Pete would laugh when he re-learned to do something simple like tie his shoes. He was shocked at how happy he was just to be able to put on his own pants. And instead of being depressed, he saw the humor in the fact that he was excited to dress himself. We would both laugh and that type of thing was what let me know that we were on our way back to a normal life —when we started laughing, together.

There was a point where I realized that I was really close to feeling like his mother and I think he was close to feeling like I was his mother. I knew enough to know that long-term, that wouldn't be good for a marriage. I hate seeing grown men treated like children by their wives and I would assume that it is certainly not a turn-on to the husbands either. During those months when I had to be Pete's caretaker (code word for "mother"), it was okay. He was helpless. But when things started to evolve, I saw it and he saw it and whatever was the least emasculating was certainly the best for both of us. So I turned the reigns over to him. That is not to say I stopped worrying.

Pete was gaining strength every day and it was a little bit hard for me to keep up. I was always worried he was going to trip and fall. Or slip in the shower. Or…..the list was endless. I tried to give him back responsibility for himself as he was ready to take it back. I think that we both waffled on those things sometimes.

Everything that I focused on was short term. Really short term. There was no long term planning, which was something Pete and I had always loved to do. It was day-by-day plans of how to get him healthier and how to offer the kids all the time I had left over. I don't think I ever once thought about Pete getting well so we could tour again, or so he could record music again. If anything, I think I assumed that he wouldn't be doing those things again. He was so deeply ill, even as he was recovering, that I didn't imagine our life would ever be the way it was before. My long-term plans went about as far as two weeks out. The upside of that is that I didn't have too much time to lament the fact that things might never be the same again. I did worry about income and how he would make a living, but as his manager I focused my energy in ways to re-market all the amazing music he'd already created and how to build a career out of never leaving town. There were a million ways to do that, and I would investigate all of them, once Pete even felt like discussing it.

So we had just returned to Nashville and within two months I was supposed to go to Aspen as co-producer of the annual John Denver Tribute Concert—the one where Pete and I had first met. I was so torn. I'd never missed one and it's one of the things I do that I look forward to most every year. But Pete was not going to be in any condition for me to leave him. At least that was my thinking at the time. But I just couldn't throw in the towel. So I kept my co-producer Mark Johnson hanging until I could make a decision. Meanwhile, I lined up a home health care nurse who lives in our neighborhood and who had helped us before Pete went to Houston.

Every day I would agonize over what was the right thing to do. At the same time, Pete was slowly becoming more self-suffi-cient. And he started to get some of his personality back—and his sense of humor. Ever so slowly. And then he said it, "I want to come to Aspen with you." What? Is he insane? Back to the high altitude scene of the crime – back to 8,000 feet altitude (7,908 to be exact). What was he thinking? He's never been a daredevil, but I think he really needed to see his bandmates, and the fans that had emotionally and financially supported us over the last year. I think he needed them to see that he was alive. Not back to himself, but alive. I also think he was a little worried about being separated from me. I told him I would just not go to

Aspen and stay home with him. But the next week during our weekly hospital visit, he asked the doctor if he could go. They were stunned. They didn't want him to go, but they didn't forbid him. Now we hadn't been anywhere but Houston and Nashville for the last six months. We would have to fly out there, which is obviously a high altitude, and then be in Aspen for a week. He was pretty firm that it was what he wanted to do and even though I tried to gently ignore his interest in going, he held the doctor's feet to the fire. They said that if he went, which they didn't really recommend, that he would have to have oxygen with him the whole time out there. He agreed. I booked the flights.

Aspen in October is absolutely beautiful, and we'd been enjoying that for 12 years up to this point. It was always a special trip there because it was where we first met and decided to work together in 1998.

Even though I looked forward to it, I was also dreading it. We decided that instead of flying directly into Aspen, we would fly into Denver and spend the night, then drive up into the mountains allowing for a slightly slower adjustment to the altitude. We only told Mark Johnson and a couple of close friends that he was coming—he wanted it to be a surprise and we also didn't want to get anyone's hopes up in case he didn't come. We also told the band that Pete wouldn't be playing since we had arranged for another musician to take his place on this year's show.

The reception from friends and fans was overwhelming. From the moment Pete got out of the car and walked into the lobby, he was embraced with hugs and tears. It was so healing for both of us. And frankly I got the same reception. People thanking me for taking such good care of him. And people who had been caregivers themselves at one time or another – sympathizing with me and encouraging me.

Of course we had to let them all know that Pete wasn't performing, but came just to be with everyone and to sit in the wings and watch his bandmates. Frankly, I knew that would never fly. Pete can't stand being in a room full of great musicians and just watching. He's going to want to play.

So, he went to rehearsal. Offered up some pointers. Played a little bit in the green room. Just generally hung out as if he was going to be on stage the next two nights. Mark Johnson was kind enough to tell Pete, "If you want to play, you can play. We'll set up a spot for you on stage." But we all decided to keep it informal.

Pete watched the first half of the concert from the wings, staring intently and keeping his oxygen on most of the time. I knew he wanted to be out there more than anything. That night after the first half of the show was over, and intermission had wound down, the curtain went up for the second half. Chris Nole, the keyboard player, did a beautiful version of John Denver's "For You." Then the rest of the band took the stage. Mark Johnson stepped up to the microphone and made a beautiful and somewhat tearful comment on Pete and his health battles over the past year. Then he introduced Pete who slowly walked out on stage and sat on a stool center stage. One of the band members handed him his guitar, and the audience went crazy. A standing ovation with a lot of fans in tears. They were stunned to see him on stage. It was a huge moment that gives me goose bumps to this day. Of course, Pete tired very, very easily, so after a couple of songs, he waved to the crowd and walked back into the wings.

The next night, with a mostly new crowd, Pete walked out in the second half to the same reception. But this time, he played the entire second half of the show. He had a huge smile on his face. As did I. This is something that we both thought we'd never get to experience again. Me in the wings watching him on stage.

After much rejoicing and visiting and overall celebrating of John Denver and Pete's life, we headed out of Aspen on a Monday morning. There was no snow yet, so instead of the usual interstate route, Pete wanted to drive out over Independence Pass via the Continental Divide. The peak altitude is 12,095 feet. At this point, who am I to argue? Pete obviously has a handle on what he can and can't do. Or he's just lacking oxygen at this point and making crazy decisions. But I tend to accommodate his wishes because he's been through hell and there's nothing I enjoy more than making him smile. So off we went in our rental car and made the 30 minute slow climb out of Aspen over the divide and back down into Denver. But at the peak – the top of the world – Pete asked me to stop the car and take a picture. He got out and walked over to the huge sign that read:

CONTINENTAL DIVIDE: ELEVATION 12,095 FEET

He said, "Take my picture." I did.

Then my sick sense of humor decided we should send it to his doctors – so we emailed it right there from the phone. Pete was all for it. I knew his sense of humor was back! Finally! He trusts his doctors implicitly but also knows that they can be very serious and stiff. He thought it was hysterical that we sent them the photo knowing they would freak out and think, "Where's his oxygen?"

Within a week I got an email from one of the nurses asking if Pete's cardiologist could use the photo in a presentation she was making? I thought about it and said, "Well, as long as it is being used in a positive way and the caption underneath doesn't read

'What an idiot!', then you are welcome to use it." The nurse laughed and said she would make sure of it.

Over the next few doctor's appointments we noticed that every doctor, every nurse, every specialist and blood taker had an 8x10, color print of the photo of Pete we sent. When they would open their folder of his medical records, the picture would be paper clipped to the inside of the folder. We got such a huge laugh out of it. We weren't sure if they were all sharing it because they were proud of their patient or if they circulated it as a "most wanted" photo of a lunatic with a VAD. Either way, we were proud that it made an impact.

On December 22, 2011, four months after we returned home from Houston, Dr. Fish dropped by for a visit. This always made us a little nervous. Frank rarely came by the house and the few times he did were when Pete was racing toward heart failure, or when there was an official invitation of a social kind. This time he asked if he could drop by. We sat and caught up for a little while, and then he slowly revealed the nature of his visit. He'd been designated to give us the news that Pete was being considered officially "non-transplantable." Keep in mind that Pete wasn't really eager to have another open heart surgery, ever. But through this entire ordeal, we had kept our eye on the prize which was….a new heart.

The decision was based on many great cardiac minds putting their thoughts on paper and nobody could guarantee a survival rate higher than 50%. That's not too good. Not good for us, and not good for the hospital and doctors. Too much risk for them. This was so depressing. I'm used to setting a goal and doing whatever it takes to reach it. It was out of my hands. Pete officially went from having a VAD that was considered a "bridge to transplant" to a "destination therapy." Meaning it's what he would have forever, however long that was.

I remember being sick for days. The usual excitement I had during the buildup for Christmas just couldn't be mustered. I didn't want to talk to anyone, or celebrate. I felt like we'd finally hit the wall. Nowhere to go. Nothing more could be done. I became pretty introspective, as did Pete. We talked it through a lot. Our practical side really comes in handy during times like these. The fact is that Pete didn't want another surgery. These days he says, "I wouldn't take a heart if they gave me one." Neither of us wanted to take the high risk of failure. We'd come too far to risk losing everything. We were so grateful that he had survived and was improving on a daily basis. So I flipped the switch and got over being sad about it. Now what?

Pete Huttlinger and Erin Morris Huttlinger

Chapter Twenty

Pete Plays Again. "Damn It"

Pete

So here we are back in Nashville after six weeks at Vanderbilt University Medical Center and a four-month stay at the Texas Heart Institute in Houston. Now what? I need to concentrate on getting healthy again. I need to decide if I'm going to try to be a serious guitar player again. But not today. I'm too tired. I'll just play a few minutes and then put the guitar down for a few days. Pick it up again and decide later. I just want some sleep.

It actually hurt to play. Physical pain runs through the fingers on my left hand. I look at myself in the mirror. The shadowy figure of myself stares back at me. The term Auschwitz victim keeps coming to me. I am one of them. Just skin and bones. It dawns on me I'm so skinny that maybe I need some meat on my fingers. Has anyone ever tried to gain weight on their fingers before? I think to myself, "It couldn't have been this bad the first time around." Then I remember that I did it after the stroke. I learned to play again. It didn't hurt that much then. So why now? Why in the world does it hurt just to press my fingers down on the strings? Often times I would shout out "Damn it!" when the pain would begin. Erin would just sit there, calmly, and say something like, "Just play for a few minutes today and then try again tomorrow." So I would play for a few minutes with no intention of picking up my guitar the next day.

It had really been closer to a year since I'd played hard like I used to. I know that I was still doing a few gigs when my heart was failing but between the gigs, at home, I wasn't playing much at all. It took too much effort to get up out of the chair and grab a guitar. Everything took too much effort.

I would go to the cardio rehab center for a little workout two times per week. That was as much as my health insurance would allow. That was okay. Two times a week there with a little supervision and then I could walk in our neighborhood or out in the park on the other days.

Erin would try to get me to play. Sometimes I would. Sometimes I wouldn't. But I did notice something. The more I did it, the easier it became. I know that sounds simple and logical now

but back then I was unable to have a coherent thought sometimes.

I was unable to play with a flat-pick after the stroke. I could
strum down. But an upstroke proved too elusive. I knew what I
was supposed to be able to do but I was unable to get my right
hand to cooperate. So I bought a little 1950 Gibson L-50 from
our friend Kim Sherman at Cotton Music in Nashville after the
stroke to play Freddie Green-style rhythm.

But now after so many months without playing, I couldn't
finger-pick either. And my left hand hurt to press the strings.
Things were not looking good. It was not easy wrapping my
head around the fact that I would no longer be a guitarist. But
my humor was intact. I would say to Erin, "Okay so I'm not a
guitar player any more. I can still work. I can sell used cars or
shoes. Or maybe I could be a lamp repairman. The possibilities
are endless."

There were many days when Erin would say to me, "Pete,
why don't you just play for a few minutes today and we'll see how
you feel tomorrow." So reluctantly, I would do as she asked.
"Damn it!" she'd hear after just a few minutes.

I tried visualization techniques. I would lie in bed at night or
in the morning and see myself playing the guitar in my mind. I
have used this technique many times over the years. If I can see it
in my mind, I can do it in reality. But there was a problem. No
matter how hard I tried, no matter how patient I was, I couldn't
see much of what I used to be able to do. I learned over time that
I was not yet ready to do those things and that was why I couldn't
yet see them in my mind. As time progressed I was able to see
more and more.

But then slowly, ever so slowly, things started to turn around.

There are several milestones I recall that were significant in my recovery as a player. Jason Shadrick from Premier Guitar Magazine asked me to do a couple of articles for him. "It's no big deal," he said. "Just record a few examples and write out the music." No big deal for you, I thought. No one knew that I couldn't play anymore. They all knew me as Pete-the-player. Not Pete-the-has-been player. But I did the first one for Jason. It went well. I just recorded a simple exercise that I could play and wrote it out.

I flash back to my teaching days years ago. I remember that I gained more than any of my students ever did by coming up with exercises for them. It was the whole process that helped me so much. Coming up with the exercise. Writing it out. Practicing the exercise to make sure I could play it better than my student. The next one I did was just a little bit more difficult. "Damn it!" was heard from the living room at home.

Our dear friend Cynthia returned for our regular Sunday get togethers. She would sing and I would struggle to play. A friend like Cynthia is rare in this world. She is a total giver. She asks for nothing. She loves to sing more than anybody I've ever known and she just wanted to help me. Friends don't get any better than that. She also has a cupcake business and she would bring over a dozen cupcakes every Sunday to help me put on a little weight.

Then one evening I got a call from my friend Jim Wood. He is a great fiddler and Jim is a black and white kind of guy. What can you do? How can you do it more? How can you do better? He's very good at looking at a situation, analyzing it and finding a way to get out of it. Jim asked how I was doing. I told him I wasn't really playing any more. I just couldn't do it. I had done one or two little gigs in town but there was nothing on the horizon. He listened to me and said, "Well, I've been thinking. I could give you some money but that won't last too long and I really think you're like me in that you'd rather earn the money for yourself rather than just have it given to you. So I've got a proposition for you. I've got five gigs booked for us to play. You get all the money and that will be my contribution to your health account." I was listening, I said. He continued, "It will be you, me, my wife Inge and our friend Hillary. You'll have to play a lot of mandolin and there's a fair amount of Bach involved but we'll also do some old-time music, Celtic tunes and fiddle tunes. What do you think?" It was like manna from heaven. It was going to be a lot of work but my friend Jim had just given me the opportunity of a lifetime. Something to work towards. A goal. "I'm in," I said.

Jim started sending me files of music to learn immediately and the first gig was six weeks away. Maybe I could do it. I began practicing harder than I had in a long time. Bach is not easy to play and it's even harder after you've had a stroke and heart failure. I drove out to his house near Shelbyville, TN several times so we could all practice together. It was tough but if they were willing, how could I not be?

We did the gigs and I was not stellar by any means. But I got through the music and I saw that maybe I could be a player again. This was just the beginning of a very long journey but I had decided to make that journey for the third time in my life. I still wanted to play the guitar.

There were more bad days than good as I taught myself to play again. But every now and then a light that had been off for so long would come on and I made progress. I would try to fingerpick something and it just wouldn't work. "Damn it!"

I would try a flat-pick and I couldn't make it hit the strings I was aiming for. "Damn it!" Then I would fingerpick something again and voila! It worked. All I needed was a little bit of success and I was off and running.

One day I was sitting in our kitchen and I was playing around with my guitar. I started thinking about a CD I had done that I humorously called *Finger Picking Wonder: The Music of Stevie Wonder.* There's a tune on there that was always very difficult for me to play even before any of my troubles. "I Wish" is a fantastic tune. I started to wonder if I could ever play that one again. I thought if I could play that, maybe I'd have a shot at the guitar. So I pulled out the music and started in again. The infectious bass line was easy enough but then I had to add the horn stabs. That actually came together rather quickly. Over the next two weeks I had the whole thing under my fingers and I was learning something about myself. I could do it for a third time. I could learn to play again. Each little success was fun again.

Aubrey Haynie's words came back to me. Maybe I wouldn't be the player I was before all this happened, but I could still play pretty darned well if I could only be patient and accept whatever gifts given to me as they were given to me.

God grant me the serenity....

For the longest time, each day would bring back something that I couldn't do the day before. As hard as that may be to believe, it is true. Some new pattern from my right hand would reveal itself. An old tune that I had played for years, and then was robbed from me, would suddenly appear. The next day it would be taken away from me again but I knew that I had done it once. I would do it again. The elusive flat-pick was the most troublesome. I couldn't make it do what I wanted. Try as I would, it just would refuse to connect with what my brain was telling it to do.

Just play a simple tune. You can do it. I'd make it three measures and drop the pick or make some horrendous mistake, grab the pick and start again.

As time progressed though, and I slowly became a guitar player again, the time between revelations increased. Instead of measuring my progress daily, it had now become weekly. Sometimes a month would go by with no noteworthy progress.

However, there were still two pieces that I used to play most every morning as part of my warm-up routine that I couldn't play anymore. The first one is called Etude #1 by Hector Villa-Lobos, and it is a great exercise for the right hand. I used to love to play it to wake up my hand. With this as your guide:

P = Pulgar = Thumb

I = Indice = Index finger

M = Medio = Middle finger

A = Anular = Ring finger

The pattern goes like this p, i, p, i, p, m, i, a, m, a, i, m, p, i, p, i. It's very fast, goes on for a couple of minutes and I couldn't even get through the pattern once.

The other piece that I was playing in my warm-up is called "El Ultimo Tremolo" by Agustin Barrios Mangore. It is a fantastic showcase for the tremolo technique and I used to be able to play it pretty darned well. I just couldn't do this one either. Now this was not a huge concern for me because I never performed either of these pieces in my concert repertoire. But they were important to me as a measuring stick for my overall progress.

The main problem with these pieces and many others was with my ring finger. It no longer had the strength or coordination to play complicated things. Patterns that were so easy I had never given any thought to in the past just wouldn't be possible —- yet.

I knew this was 100% related to the stroke and had nothing to do with heart failure. But at times I would sit and blame it on both. Then just as soon, I would laugh at the insanity of the situation. A little voice inside of me would speak up from time to time. "You cannot blame something on a stroke or heart failure any more than you can blame your mother for the size of your shoes or the length of your hair. Laying blame never does anyone any good. You have to reach inside of yourself and find that strength to move on, on your own. You have to remember to laugh a lot at yourself and with those around you. Because without laughter, life is nothing. You must not be afraid of crying. Tears are a great healer. With each tear we shed we become stronger, more complete. And in between the laughter and the tears there is time to try again to be a player. Sometimes it works and sometimes it doesn't." More often now it does.

Chapter Twenty-One

The Marathon

Pete

About a month, or maybe five weeks, after we arrived back home in Nashville I began a rehab program at Vanderbilt's Dayani Center for Health & Wellness. It was a great place for me to begin my long journey back to some kind of healthfulness. I so wanted to be self-sufficient again and the staff there was encouraging and friendly in their approach. They knew that I couldn't lift any more than about five pounds and I couldn't walk very far or very fast so their work was not going to be easy.

That October I weighed in at 135 pounds on my first visit. The first thing I did there was a test where I was to walk as far as I could in six minutes. I made it less than 1,000 feet. The last time I did the six-minute walk test on April 10, 2012, I clocked 1,960 feet, which is just over 1/3 of a mile. Staff at rehab centers are a lot like doctors in that the way they respond to questions. Never a straight answer in the affirmative or the negative. Always leave you wondering just a little bit. So I was never sure how I rated compared to a "normal" person. But I suppose that doesn't matter. I knew how I was doing.

I had worked out a lot throughout my life from the time I was thirteen years-old and back from the hospital after my first open heart surgery. The first time I walked in the house my brother Frank, who was all of fifteen years-old, pointed to a set of weights and a bench in the middle of the living room and proclaimed, "Okay Pete, we'll give you two weeks to rest up and then you're hitting the weights." My brothers didn't want me to wimp out on them and I guess lifting weights was as good a way as any to see that didn't happen. Mom was kind enough to buy the weights and the bench. Two weeks later I started lifting. Just the bar at first. No weights. By the end of the summer I was bench-pressing four sets of four repetitions of 70 pounds. By the time I was a junior in high school I was bench-pressing 185 pounds. A little more than 30 pounds above my total body weight.

I'd worked out during high school in California but when we moved to North Carolina I was told I couldn't use the weight room at the school because I was not on the football team. That's when I began running.

I thought I knew all about weight lifting and proper technique but I was soon to learn that I only knew things a healthy person could do. I was no longer in that group. I was a man who could not lift much or walk far. This is where the well-trained staff at a good rehab center earns its keep. They knew that my entire body was compromised and put a plan together to work all of me. Not just cardio, which is what I thought I was going there for. I had to lift two-pound weights in each hand straight out in front of me, hold them in place and then release them slowly. The first set of repetitions was always the easiest but by the third or fourth set, I was really struggling. I quickly graduated to three-pound weights but the leap to the big daddies, the five-pounders, proved too elusive for quite some time.

Then I would get on a lifting machine for my leg muscles. This was pretty gratifying because there were numbers that I recognized from the old days. The only difference was these numbers, 40 and 50 pounds used to be lifted by my upper body and now it was all I could do to lift them with the biggest muscles in my body, my legs. Not to worry. At least it wasn't two and three pounds.

Then after legs I would get on a sit-down stationary bicycle. Ten minutes of that for my heart and I was done. "See y'all next time," I'd shout out to the trainers and I'd head home for a nap.

But then as the weeks progressed, my body began responding to the twice-weekly workouts. I stopped doing the bicycle and got on the treadmill. A mile.

Hallelujah! Then we added the elliptical machine. That one's a real doosy. It works your legs, heart and a little bit of your upper body when done properly. It was really a tough challenge for me particularly because you can change the resistance on it and I liked the fact that it had so much digital information coming off the machine. I could see how far I'd gone, at what pace, how many calories I'd burned and lots of other useful information that a patient and his/her trainer needs to measure improvement. But I liked the no-impact part of it best and so that was added to my routine.

Now after five or six weeks I was feeling improvement. I had a regular routine down: Lift weights, do the elliptical machine, do the treadmill, stretch and go home.

Around this time I heard about the marathon. I had always wanted to walk the Country Music Marathon (a full marathon is 26.2 miles but walkers do half of it or 13.1 miles). But I had always been working.

It was coming up in April 2012 and it was still only October or November of 2011. I mentioned to my trainer that I wanted to walk the half-marathon that was coming up. He didn't really look me in the eye when he said rather flippantly, "Yeah, right." He didn't think I could do it. Those two words were a wakeup call and a challenge to me.

There are two great motivators in my life. One is to make fun of me and the other is to not believe in me. He had just done both.

I remember going home that day and telling Erin that I wanted to walk the half-marathon that was coming up the following April. She immediately said, "Okay, let's do it!" I can always count on Erin to back me up.

Erin

Pete and I had started walking a lot in the park. Some days he would last 20 minutes walking. Some days we would make it about 10 minutes. But each day he got stronger and stronger and before we knew it, we were walking a mile. The weather was getting cold, but we'd bundle up and get outside. Pete loves the outdoors and just being there made him feel better. I think he started to see light at the end of his tunnel. I think we both did. He was smiling a lot more, and starting to joke. Just being in his natural environment was bringing him out of his shell. He was getting cardiac rehabilitation through Vanderbilt, but he soon outgrew it. Then it hit him. He had always wanted to walk a half-marathon. Since we had first met in 1998, Pete had mentioned to me that he wanted to walk the annual Country Music Marathon in Nashville that takes place in late April. Now he got his sights set on it again. Talk about putting pressure on me. I don't think I'd ever thought about walking a half-marathon, but if my 130 pound husband, whose heart is run primarily by a machine can do it, how could I say no. So we agreed in November of that year, that come April 28 we would walk the Country Music Marathon – and it would be exactly one year since he was life-flighted from Nashville to Houston.

So again, we had a mission.

Having a goal has been such a key part of every step of our journey. Whether it was a short term goal (keep Pete alive), or a long-term goal (walk a half-marathon), I've always had to keep my eye on something. It's more than just having a purpose. My purpose is to be a good wife, daughter and mom, but I could just swim around in those large concepts. I need a target to hit. That is one reason that Pete and I have always been a wonderful match. We like having a reason to push forward, to jump out of bed every day with great excitement, and make to do lists.

Pete was a new man with this marathon on the horizon. He enlisted family, friends and fans to "walk" with him, either in person or in their own hometowns. We were focused and looked forward.

Pete

Erin and I began walking in Percy Warner Park near our home. Dave from the coffee club is quite a walker and he told us of a few different length walks and we were off with a mission in mind. Now remember, I wasn't really working much other than trying to learn to play the guitar again, the occasional gig and of course, Cynthia would be over on Sundays to sing for me. So I had nothing else to do but concentrate on my health and getting healthier. I had been blessed beyond belief with all the money that was raised on our behalf to help cover a mountain of medical and living expenses. So without that worry hanging over me, my new full-time job was to get healthy.

We quickly got up to two miles. Up and down the roads. Winter was approaching quickly and Erin doesn't like the cold weather nearly as much as I do but what could she really say? I was committed so she sort of had to… God bless her. Then we added a mile. Three miles! "Ten more to go and we've got us a half of a marathon sweetheart."

Sometime in January we hit five miles. I wasn't walking fast but I was walking. Not one year prior I was unable to walk across my living room and now I was walking five miles. Every day we would walk I would feel a great sense of accomplishment.

Now I was still going to the Dayani Center two times per week. Lifting weights and working out harder and harder on the elliptical machine and the treadmill. I would go faster and measure my improvement. I was getting stronger and faster and I could see it all right before my eyes.

Around this time I began soliciting friends and family from around the world to walk a half marathon with me. They didn't have to come to Nashville to do it. They could do it wherever they chose. Many folks from as far away as Pennsylvania and California, to Germany and England said they were in. I was excited now, and even had a group on Facebook called Walking With Pete.

The trainer who unknowingly inspired me to do the walk was now on board with me. I was talking about it every time I went in there and I was working out hard. He would say, "Man, you're really gonna' do this aren't you?" Then he'd say, "Man, I'm gonna to be there at the finish line waiting for you. I'm gonna' be there for you!" I had won him over and I was pumped. He was going to be there at the finish line to see me complete the single hardest task I'd ever undertaken.

I tried to recruit some of my fellow Dayani Center members to walk with me. We were all pretty sick but the way I saw it, without a goal, we were going to stay sick. "C'mon are you in? Would you like to walk a half marathon? How about a portion of it? How about one mile or half a mile? Can I count on you to commit for any of it?" You'd have thought I was an alien. The response I got was not good. Most of them just looked at me like I was nuts. There was one woman, however. Her name was Norma. She was fun and excited about life. I enjoyed talking with her when we would do the treadmill together. I told her of my plans and she was interested. I had her. She was in. We walked five miles one day together up and down Belle Meade Boulevard. But that was it. One walk and she had some back pain so she was out.

I asked my trainer if he was interested in walking with me.

Nope. He had a leg injury from a recent run. His wife was going to run the half marathon so he'd "be there" for me at the end of the race.

I contacted my family. My sister T was in. Brother Frank – in. Cousin Colleen – hippest, partying-est, coolest cousin that ever was was in! Having Colleen on board was a major coup. If she was in, she could recruit folks like no one else. Cousin Cath and her husband John were in. Dr. Frank Fish – in! Erin's brother Jason and his girlfriend Jewel – in. Things were shaping up nicely.

Then the unthinkable happened.

We were using a schedule put together by Coffee Club Dave. Turns out he was a serious marathoner before his knees got so bad. He put a plan together for us so that we would gradually increase our distance and it wouldn't kill us on the day of the race. (And I use the term "race" very loosely. My goal was to finish in under four hours.) I had been training pretty hard in the hills on pavement only. Since the stroke had left me a little weak on the right side of my body, I had been favoring my left leg. A lot. I noticed a bump on my leg. No worries. I had lots of bumps. But this one was different. And it hurt like the dickens when I would stop to rest but not when I walked. So I kept on walking. After two weeks I went to Vanderbilt to get it checked out. The heart doctor that I saw was an ex runner and he looked at it and said, "Well, I know that it's not a blood clot. But I don't know what it is."

So I went to see Dr. Paul Parsons, an orthopedist at Vanderbilt. This was nine weeks before the race. He took one look at my leg and said, "I can tell you what happened. You broke your leg." "I broke my leg?" I said astonished. "How in the hell could that happen?" He said he sees it all the time leading up to the race. "I broke my damned leg? After all I've been through? A stroke. Heart failure. I'm well on my way to getting back in shape and now you're telling me I broke my goddamned leg?" It was no longer a leg. I never referred to it without "goddamned" in front of it. It's not a term I use loosely but I was so angry I thought God had surely damned my leg. After viewing the x-ray, Dr. Parsons said I would not be walking the marathon. It was just a stress fracture but it was a broken leg as far as he was concerned. He gave me a brace to wear for six weeks, told me I could do some no-impact machines but no, I would not be walking the race unless I wanted him to operate and put a metal rod in my leg.

I was pissed off and Erin knew it. After all I'd been through over the past year, the stroke, the heart failure, I had never been this angry. I had been incredibly frustrated but not angry until that moment. Erin put me in my corner and Dr. Parsons in his corner and did her magic. He eventually agreed that if he saw enough improvement with my leg in six weeks, he'd clear me to walk the marathon.

I went back to my usual docs at Vanderbilt and teased the ex-runner/cardiologist because he couldn't diagnose a broken leg. There's a real art to specializing in medicine but really, you, an ex-runner, can't recognize a broken leg? Isn't that in Doctoring 101? He left Vanderbilt shortly after that. Although I'm sure it didn't have anything to do with my leg, I still feel bad for teasing him. But hey….

Meanwhile I sent a text to Dr. Fish. It said, "I broke my dog-gone leg." He misinterpreted my text just a wee bit. He tried to call me but my ringer was off. He phoned Erin and asked about me. She said, "Yes, he broke his leg. Can you believe that kind of bad luck? He's out at the store. I'll tell him you phoned." "Oh," he said, "he's at the store? He's not lying in a field with a broken leg?" He had apparently alerted the team at Vanderbilt that I was on my way in. He had pictured me with a busted femur coming out of my upper thigh. He told Erin that he would have to go. He needed to make a phone call. He called off the team.

So me and my broken leg went back to the Dayani Center for some low impact workouts. I had to keep working my heart as much as I could. I had gone too far to lose it all just because of a "damned broken leg."

I announced via Facebook that our venture was likely over. Sent word out to Colleen, T, Frank, Cath. The race was off as far as I was concerned. Everyone offered words of encouragement but I was pretty down at that point. I really thought I was being tested and wasn't really up for another test. I was pissed off and fighting a little bit of depression.

But I did the only thing I knew how to do. I kept at it. What was the alternative? There really wasn't one. Sit on the couch and sulk? That's really not my cup of tea.

Three weeks before the marathon I went back to visit Dr. Parsons. He cleared me and sent me off with a warning, "Just get this out of your system and then just walk a couple of miles a day. I don't want to see you back in here."

Three weeks to go. I hadn't done any distance in six weeks. Could I do it? Could Erin do it? We walked two miles the first three or four days. Then we quickly got to three and within a week we were back to five miles. We took one day off each week. The schedule Dave had set up for us was out the window. It no longer applied. We had to get in a lot of miles in a short amount of time.

Then all of a sudden it was here. April 28, 2012. On April 29,

2011 I was life-flighted out of Nashville, TN to Houston, TX. — unable to walk across a street, a room and eventually unable to get out of bed for almost two months. Now here we were one year later to the day. We were going to see this thing through. We were going to walk the Country Music Marathon.

Frank, T, Cath, John, Eric, Dr. Fish, Jason, Jewel and about 31,000 of our newest friends walked, ran, hoola-hooped, wheel-chaired, or crawled across that finish line with Erin and I.

Our friends in West Virginia and Germany walked it with us in their respective places. It was so gratifying to know that so many folks decided to do something for their own health on that day.

I was looking for my trainer from the Dayani Center but I couldn't find him. I figured that was because he was just lost in the crowd. So I sent him an e-mail that evening. He responded that he wasn't there when I finished because his wife had finished earlier and they went home. Went home? What happened to, "Man, I'm gonna' be there for you!" I was crushed to say the least. The guy who had not believed in me and made fun of me and who then turned completely around and was "gonna' be there" for me was in the end a no-show. He just couldn't be bothered to stay another hour or so to see me finish.

That night we had a big cookout at our house. Everyone that walked the marathon with us, and other friends, joined us. Eric manned the grill. Dr. Fish and I played music and Eric joined us when the chicken was finished grilling. James played piano. We drank a lot of beer. We were all pretty tired and by ten o'clock the party was over and we were sleeping hard.

I went back to the Dayani Center only two more times. I couldn't work out with my trainer any longer. I was so hurt by him I couldn't even look him in the eye. I thought that as much good as he'd done for me physically, he'd just undone in my spirit. I don't know if he realized the power of one. One person. But he had it and he blew it. He had the power to make me feel like I could do this. He had the power to motivate me. But he lacked the will to see it through. I can guarantee he's not had another patient who has been through what I've been through and then completed a half marathon. But I did it, ultimately without his help or encouragement. I had my own team around me and together we did it.

I thought that I would be better off at a regular workout club so I went back to the neighborhood's Jewish Community Center where we had been members for so long before all hell (health) broke loose. I thought it was better for me to be around people who were healthy and working out hard than to be around folks who were just barely putting effort into getting healthy.

Not long after the marathon Dr. Fish came by. We sat and had a couple of beers together. He told me that he'd done some research and found that I was the only documented recipient of a heart pump who had walked a half marathon! I was not surprised but I was happy. Happy to be the first, but hopefully just that—the first. I would like to see everyone who gets a chance at life, as I have, get up, get out of bed, go for a walk. You don't have to have as lofty a goal as I did but set yourself a goal just the same and remember you can do it. Just don't accept "no" as an answer. Be willing to accept defeat but then build on it. Get up and try again tomorrow… or later on today. YOU CAN DO IT.

Chapter Twenty-Two

"Don't Just Live, Live Well"

Erin

The year 2012 was a building year. I don't know if we knew what we were building up to, but we were building. Building stamina, building our relationship, building health, building stability with the kids, building our careers. And then one day it hit me. I felt normal. And that everything didn't revolve around Pete's health. Slowly but surely

227

Pete began playing his guitar seriously. He worked diligently to re-build his skills. He was meticulous about it. He re-built himself from the ground up. I tried to be encouraging but not overly excited. I tried to be supportive and would cheer him on without hyping him or telling him he sounded great when he didn't. Honesty is what our entire relationship has been built upon beginning back in 1998 when we started working together.

I started to bring up some of the things we used to talk about on a daily basis. Recording. Live performances. Teaching. Even traveling, which made us both terribly nervous. These ideas didn't seem so far-fetched anymore. I began pulling out my little green spiral notebook. The one that signified we were having a meeting. It was dusty, but we were ready. We had gotten into a rhythm of doctor's checkups and giving blood for lab work, but those things didn't consume our every waking hour any longer.

We returned to our Bruegger's coffee club gang. That was our symbol of "normal." Remember the tv show "Cheers" when any given character would walk through the door? They would be acknowledged by the whole gang, but not overly so. That was our group. Everyone was happy to see us, but didn't make us feel self-conscious.

My brain was foggy and out of practice but we were both excited to slowly slip back into our normal patterns of planning and executing, and looking forward to our future because we finally believed we had a future.

So much has changed over the last couple of years, but in a big picture way everything is back to normal. Our version of normal. It's been so exciting working together in the way that we used to. We've started touring again and although we don't tour to the extent we did, we're working just as much. Historically,

Pete and I usually traveled together, we now always travel together. We have a lot of extra baggage, literally, because of all the battery packs, charging stations, bandages, medicines, etc… Pete isn't supposed to lift heavy bags or crates anymore—and these are obviously things that can't be avoided when touring. So we do it together. I'm there 100% of the time, as roadie and as a traveling nurse should an emergency arise. I'm there to change his bandages regularly—and even though we've tried to figure out a way for him to do that for himself, I think that's an intimacy we share and enjoy. He's the willing patient and I can still care for him just a little bit. Other than that he is completely self-sufficient, and that's important to him. But mostly I'm just traveling as his wife. We cherish all of our time.

We've also created a lot of new income streams. One that we enjoy tremendously is our Pete Huttlinger Guitar Camps that we host in our home. Pete teaches, I cook and we meet a lot of interesting folks.

One of the most exciting and important things we are now also doing is speaking engagements. We have a speech titled Don't Just Live, Live Well, and it's a multi-media event that includes a lot of stories, pictures and music. It tells the story that we've told here and not only are we encouraging everyday folks, and people with medical conditions, we find that we are really inspiring the medical community. So many surgeons, doctors, nurses and nurse practitioners have come up to us following our speeches. They crave some positive reinforcement that the work they are doing means something. All their patients disappear after they are released from the hospital. They don't get the opportunity to see how they fare or how they go into the world and do good things with the gifts they've been given. More often they see patients that go back home and spend the rest of their life sitting on the couch and watching TV. It makes them happy, they say, to see someone thriving, not just living.

Once, after a visit back to Texas Heart Institute, Pete gave a brief concert for all the nurses and doctors involved in cardiology. It was the first time that a lot of them even realized Pete was an entertainer. Dr. Frazier's partner, Dr. Billy Cohn, also happens to be a musician and he sat in on a couple of tunes with Pete. It was a wonderful concert and there was a lot of joy and feelings of success on all our parts.

Dr. Frazier pulled me aside after the concert. It was the first time we'd had a non-medical conversation. As a pioneer in the invention of artificial hearts and cardiac assist devices, Dr. Frazier has had a lot of successes and failures. Failure is all part of the field of science and invention. He told me that over his decades in surgical trial and error with these devices, he lost a lot of patients initially. In fact, he told me that after the first 22 patients didn't survive, he was asked if he was going to give up. He replied to them saying "Of course I'm not giving up. These 22 people have given their lives and it has to be for a reason." He then told me that Pete was the perfect example of what he'd been working towards all these years. Someone that didn't just survive, but someone that thrived! It was the first time I'd ever seen him beam with such a big smile. Then he handed us a note. It read, "Pete, Don't just live, live well. Bud Frazier"

We've adopted that as our motto and everywhere we go we try to share that message. "Don't just live, live well."

We've been enveloped by so much good fortune and love from so many people. It has enhanced our lives and made us excited about every single day that we wake up and pursue our dreams. These experiences have made us even more aware and grateful. There are so many things that we want to do together as we grow old, even though we don't know how old that will be.

We just operate as if we'll both live to be 100 and who knows, maybe we will.

Epilogue

"You'll like him. Nice guy. Musician." That was the understated but totally accurate description of Pete Huttlinger made by his previous cardiologist when he referred Pete to me for assessment and treatment of his arrhythmias. Seventeen years later, Pete has amazed me many times over and continues to do so. His story is a series of inspirational themes. As a child and teen, he overcame complex cyanotic heart disease to develop into a highly regarded musician in this town of musicians. He refused to be relegated to his easy chair, choosing instead to hike the Rocky Mountains and wade through trout streams across the US. Faced with what would have been a debilitating stroke, he conducted a private bedside master performance to his Neuro ICU team three days after the stroke occurred. After receiving his VAD (Ventricular Assist Device), he didn't settle for returning to daily living. Instead, he walked a full half-marathon. Time and again, he has displayed a lust for living that's far beyond his expected limitations rather than letting himself be defined by them.

Congenital heart disease of varying severity affects approximately eight out of every 1,000 infants born. Pete was born with a complex heart defect known as "congenitally corrected transposition of the great arteries," combined with a hole in the heart (ventricular septal defect) and an abnormal valve which limited the amount of blood flow to his lungs. As if all these afflictions were not severe enough, they were made all the more complex by the fact that his heart, major arteries and veins, and other vital organs are reversed in his body.

When he first came to us, there were already concerning signs about his cardiac status. While the imaging tests suggested he might soon need to be considered for a heart transplant, his lifestyle suggested he was nowhere near ready. As time wore on and gradually took its toll on his heart, he continued to exercise and do everything possible to stave off the eventuality of end-stage heart failure. When faced with the reality of depending on a mechanical device for his survival, he refused to abandon his "can do" approach to life.

Pete has lived his entire life outpacing everyone else's expectations for him and continues to do so today. All of us have had bad days. Many of us have faced hardships that seemed insurmountable. Some of us have even been on the brink of death with so few options. However, few of us have displayed the notion of "living each day to the fullest" like this remarkable man.

Pete has certainly had help—from dedicated physicians and skilled musical instructors and mentors to the unwavering support of his family and many friends.

In his wife, Erin, he has found a like-minded partner. Together, they have navigated the rocks in the stream and focused on overcoming and managing problems instead of than having their lives and relationship defined by them. Through it all, Pete has maintained his humor, his humility, and his genuine sense of caring for others. He has given back far more than he has been given, many times over.

I have cared for many adult patients born with comparably

complex cardiac defects who have lowered their goals and expectations, if not given up altogether. A few, like Pete, refuse to accept other's limitations or fall victim to self-pity. They have become lawyers, physicians, teachers, politicians, rodeo riders, and, in this case, an extraordinary guitar player and human being. How Pete lives his life is relevant to us all.

Nice guy. Musician. Inspiration. Friend. Teacher. That about sums it up.

— Frank Fish, M.D.
Vanderbilt University Medical Center
Professor of Pediatrics
Associate Professor of Medicine
Director of Pediatric and Adult Congenital Electrophysiology

**For a free MP3 copy of the song,
"Things Are Looking Up,"
go to Pete's website www.petehuttlinger.com,
purchase the song and enter
JOINED AT THE HEART
in the coupon code. It will be free.**

Music by Pete Huttlinger available at
www.petehuttlinger.com

ALBUMS:
Catch & Release
Naked Pop
The Need
The Santa Rita Connection
Things Are Looking Up
Fingerpicking Wonder
The Black Swan
Hymns For Guitar Vols. I & II
First Light – A Pete Huttlinger Christmas
McGuire's Landing

For concert or speaking bookings contact:

Erin Morris
SANTA RITA ARTIST MANAGEMENT
erin@morrispr.biz

www.petehuttlingerspeaks.com

.

Pete Huttlinger is one of the world's most awe-inspiring acoustic guitar players. His imaginative arrangements, spellbinding musicality and riotous sense of humor have dazzled audiences from Los Angeles to Milan, both in his role as a solo artist and as lead guitarist for such headliners as John Denver, John Oates (of Hall & Oates) and LeAnn Rimes. He has played Carnegie Hall and Eric Clapton's Crossroads Festival three times each. He's also recorded and produced more than a dozen albums.

Erin Huttlinger, Pete's wife, is a veteran publicist and artist-development specialist. At RCA Records, she enhanced and spotlighted the careers of Kenny Rogers, Dolly Parton, Charley Pride, Alabama, Waylon Jennings, The Judds, Roy Rogers and Keith Whitley, among others. As an independent publicist, she has helmed publicity campaigns for such stars as Vince Gill, LeAnn Rimes, Ralph Stanley, Martina McBride, Merle Haggard, Ricky Skaggs, Steve Wariner and The Time Jumpers.

In addition to Pete's concert tours, he and Erin also offer inspirational multimedia presentations that chronicle their triumphs over Pete's seemingly insurmountable medical problems to enable him to continue performing. It's called "Don't Just Live, Live Well."

CPSIA information can be obtained at www.ICGtesting.com
Printed in the USA
LVOW11s0341310116

472961LV00004B/5/P